Innovative Approaches on Cavovarus Deformity: Thinking Outside of the Box

Editor

ALESSIO BERNASCONI

FOOT AND ANKLE CLINICS

www.foot.theclinics.com

Consulting Editor
CESAR DE CESAR NETTO

December 2023 • Volume 28 • Number 4

ELSEVIER

1600 John F. Kennedy Boulevard • Suite 1800 • Philadelphia, Pennsylvania, 19103-2899

http://www.theclinics.com

FOOT AND ANKLE CLINICS Volume 28, Number 4
December 2023 ISSN 1083-7515, ISBN-978-0-443-13055-7

Editor: Megan Ashdown
Developmental Editor: Anita Chamoli

Foot and Ankle Clinics (ISSN 1083-7515) is published quarterly by Elsevier, Inc., 360 Park Avenue South, New York, NY 10010-1710. Months of issue are March, June, September, and December. Periodicals postage paid at New York, NY, and additional mailing offices. Subscription price per year is $362.00 (US individuals), $635.00 (US institutions), $100.00 (US students), $389.00 (Canadian individuals), $762.00 (Canadian institutions), $100.00 (Canadian students), $504.00 (international individuals), $762.00 (international institutions), and $215.00 (international students). To receive student/resident rate, orders must be accompanied by name of affiliated institution, date of term, and the *signature* of program/residency coordinator on institution letterhead. Orders will be billed at individual rate until proof of status is received. Foreign air speed delivery is included in all *Clinics* subscription prices. All prices are subject to change without notice. **POSTMASTER:** Send address changes to *Foot and Ankle Clinics*, Elsevier Health Sciences Division, Subscription Customer Service, 3251 Riverport Lane, Maryland Heights, MO 63043. **Customer Service: 1-800-654-2452 (US and Canada). From outside of the United States and Canada, call 314-447-8871. Fax: 314-447-8029. E-mail: JournalsCustomerService-usa@ elsevier.com (for print support); JournalsOnlineSupport-usa@elsevier.com (for online support).**

Reprints. For copies of 100 or more, of articles in this publication, please contact the Commercial Reprints Department, Elsevier Inc., 360 Park Avenue South, New York, NY 10010-1710. Tel.: 212-633-3874; Fax: 212-633-3820; E-mail: reprints@elsevier.com.

Contributors

CONSULTING EDITOR

CESAR DE CESAR NETTO, MD, PhD
Assistant Professor, Director of the Orthopedic Functional Imaging Research Laboratory (OFIRL), Department of Orthopedics and Rehabilitation, University of Iowa, Carver College of Medicine, Iowa City, Iowa, USA; Division of Orthopedic Foot and Ankle Surgery, Department of Orthopedic Surgery, Duke University, Duke University Medical Center, Durham, North Carolina, USA

EDITOR

ALESSIO BERNASCONI, MD, PhD, FEBOT
Foot and Ankle Orthopaedic and Trauma Surgeon, Department of Public Health, Trauma and Orthopaedic Unit, University Federico II of Naples, Naples, Italy

AUTHORS

AHMED KHALIL ATTIA, MD, PGDipClinEd
Department of Orthopaedic Surgery, University of Pittsburgh, Pittsburgh, Pennsylvania, USA

GASPARD AUBOYNEAU, MD
Pole de santé Léonard de Vinci, Chambray les Tours, France

JORDANNA MARIA PEREIRA BERGAMASCO, MD
Foot and Ankle Group, Santa Casa de Misericórdia de São Paulo, São Paulo, Brazil

ALESSIO BERNASCONI, MD, PhD, FEBOT
Foot and Ankle Orthopaedic and Trauma Surgeon, Department of Public Health, Trauma and Orthopaedic Unit, University Federico II of Naples, Naples, Italy

BERNHARD DEVOS BEVERNAGE, MD
Foot and Ankle Surgeon, Department of Orthopaedics, Ghent University Hospital, Ghent, Belgium; Department of Orthopaedics, Foot and Ankle Institute, Brussels, Belgium

JEAN M. BRILHAULT, MD, PhD
Centre Cheville & Pied, Clinique St Léonard, Trélazé, France

KRISTIAN BUEDTS, MD
Foot and Ankle Surgeon, Foot and Ankle Unit, Orthopedics and Traumatology Department, ZNA Middelheim, Antwerpen, Belgium; Gewrichtskliniek, Berchem, Belgium

ARNE BURSSENS, MD, PhD
Foot and Ankle Surgeon, Department of Orthopaedics, Ghent University Hospital, Ghent, Belgium

INÊS CASAIS, MD
Serviço de Ortopedia, Orthopedics and Traumatology Department, Centro Hospitalar de Vila Nova de Gaia e Espinho, Vila Nova de Gaia, Portugal

MARCO TÚLIO COSTA, MD
Foot and Ankle Group, Santa Casa de Misericórdia de São Paulo, São Paulo, Brazil

LOUIS DAGNEAUX, MD, PhD
Orthopaedic Surgeon, Senior Consultant, Head, Department of Orthopedic Surgery, Lower Limb Surgery Unit, Univ Montpellier, Laboratoire de mécanique et génie civil (LMGC), CNRS, Montpellier University of Excellence (MUSE), Montpellier, France

PIETER D'HOOGHE, MD, PhD
Aspetar Orthopaedic and Sports Medicine Hospital, Doha, Qatar

VÉRONIQUE DARCEL DARCEL, MD
Department of Orthopaedics, Maison de Santé Protestante de Bordeaux Bagatelle, Bordeaux, France

ELENA DELMASTRO, MD
Università Vita-Salute San Raffaele, Milano, Italy

CAOS France
CAOS (Computer Assisted Orthopaedic Surgery) France, Société Française de Chirurgie orthopédique et Traumatologie (SOFCOT), Paris, France

ANIL HALDAR, MBBS, FRCS (Orth)
Foot and Ankle Fellow, Department of Foot and Ankle Surgery, Royal National Orthopaedic Hospital, London, United Kingdom

ASHRAF T. HANTOULY, MD, MSc
Department of Orthopedic Surgery, Hamad Medical Corporation, Doha, Qatar

KHALID HASAN, MD, MPH
Department of Orthopaedic Surgery, Virginia Commonwealth University, Richmond, Virginia, USA

VENU KAVARTHAPU, FRCS(Orth)
Consultant Orthopaedic Surgeon, King's College Hospital, Denmark Hill, London, United Kingdom

THOMAS LORCHAN LEWIS, BSc (Hons), MBChB (Hons) MFSTEd FRCS (Tr & Orth)
King's Foot and Ankle Unit, Department of Orthopaedics, King's College Hospital NHS Foundation Trust, London, United Kingdom

FRANÇOIS LINTZ, MD, MSc, FEBOT
Ramsay Santé Clinique de l'Union, Centre de Chirurgie de la Cheville et du Pied, Saint Jean, France

JULIE MATHIEU, MD
Orthopaedic Surgeon, Senior Consultant, Department of Orthopedic Surgery, Lower Limb Surgery Unit, Univ Montpellier, Montpellier, France

MAX P. MICHALSKI, MD, MSc
Assistant Professor, Department of Orthopaedic Surgery, Cedars-Sinai Medical Center, Los Angeles, California, USA

CONOR MORAN, MD
Centre Osteo Articulaires des Cèdres, Echirolles, France

NOÉ DE MARCHI NETO, MD
Foot and Ankle Group, Santa Casa de Misericórdia de São Paulo, São Paulo, Brazil

GLENN B. PFEFFER, MD
Professor, Department of Orthopaedic Surgery, Cedars-Sinai Medical Center, Los Angeles, California, USA

BARBARA PICLET-LEGRÉ, MD
Department of Orthopaedics, Centre du pied, La Ciotat, Marseille, France

ROBBIE RAY, MB, ChB, ChM (T&O), FRCSed(Tr & Orth), FEBOT
King's Foot and Ankle Unit, King's College Hospital NHS Foundation Trust, London, United Kingdom

LOUIS RONY, MD, PhD
Département de Chirurgie Osseuse, CHU-Angers, Angers, France

ANNY STEENWERCKX, MD
Orthopaedics and Traumatology Department, AZ Diest, Diest, Belgium

MANFRED THOMAS, MD
Department of Foot and Ankle Surgery, Hessingpark Clinic, Augsburg, Germany

MADHU TIRUVEEDHULA, FRCSGlasg(Orth)
Consultant Orthopaedic Surgeon, Mid and South Essex Foundation NHS Trust, Basildon Hospital, Nethermayne, Basildon, United Kingdom

YVES TOURNÉ, MD, PhD
Centre Osteo Articulaires des Cèdres, Echirolles, France

MATTHEW JAMES WELCK, MBBS, BSc, MSc, FRCS(Orth)
Department of Foot and Ankle Surgery, Royal National Orthopaedic Hospital, London, United Kingdom

RAZI ZAIDI, BSc (Hons), MD FRCS (Tr & Orth)
King's Foot and Ankle Unit, King's College Hospital NHS Foundation Trust, London, United Kingdom

Editorial Advisory Board

Contents

The Role Of Minimally Invasive Osteotomies In Cavovarus Foot Reconstruction: Detailed Technique And Evidence For Procedures

Razi Zaidi, Thomas Lorchan Lewis, and Robbie Ray

Percutaneous correction of cavus foot deformity can be achieved with satisfactory correction of foot anatomy and biomechanics. Surgical management of cavovarus foot reconstruction is an individualized combination of surgical procedures designed to correct deformity. Minimally invasive procedures using high-torque low-speed burr can facilitate large deformity correction without extensive soft tissue stripping. This article presents the operative technique for percutaneous cavus foot correction including a lateralizing calcaneal osteotomy and proximal first ray osteotomy. However, methodologically robust evidence to support this procedure is lacking at present, and further research, particularly, focusing on long-term clinical outcomes and follow-up is required.

Cavovarus Deformity: Why Weight-Bearing Computed Tomography Should Be a First-Line Imaging Modality

François Lintz and Alessio Bernasconi

Cavovarus foot is a complex three-dimensional deformity, which includes a wide range of clinical conditions from subtle deformities to disabling feet. In this article, the authors discuss the role of weight-bearing computed tomography, which might enable to avoid double imaging (radiographs + tomography) in patients for which a detailed osteoarticular assessment is required, with the advantage to obtain tomographic images in standing position and a reduction of radiation exposure.

Is Subtle Cavovarus a Problem for Athletes?

Ashraf T. Hantouly, Ahmed Khalil Attia, Khalid Hasan, and Pieter D'Hooghe

Cavovarus or high-arched foot is a common foot deformity that occurs due to the disruption of the foot-driven equilibrium between the first metatarsal, fifth metatarsal, and the heel. This imbalance leads to an increase in the foot's normal plantar concavity. Cavovarus deformity ranges from a mild and flexible malalignment to a fixed, complex, and severe deformation. Subtle cavovarus foot, the mild form of the cavus foot, was first described by Manoli and colleagues.

Toes Deformities in Cavovarus: How to Approach Them

Barbara Piclet-Legré and Véronique Darcel

Sagittal lesser toe deformities (LTD) are the most common in cavus foot. They are mainly the result of muscular imbalance between intrinsic and extrinsic muscles. Surgery is the second-line treatment if medical treatment fails.

The aim of the present study was to provide an update on classification and surgical management of LTD in cavus foot including percutaneous procedures with a special focus on sagittal deformities. Joint sparing procedures are preferred for reducible LTD, whereas lesser toe fusions are used for rigid one in association with tendon transfer or percutaneous procedures depending of surgeon's experience and patient's clinical examination.

In order to understand the relation among ankle instability, peroneal disorders, and cavovarus deformity, it is mandatory to clarify the different stages of those disorders and also to put them into relation to each other. Finally, we need to take the patients compliance and expectations into consideration to define the individually right way of treatment.

When a patient presents with posterior heel pain on the background of a cavovarus foot, there are many different aspects to take into account. The morphology of the foot and the specific cause of the patient's pain lead the practitioner to alter the treatment appropriately. Some patients should only receive physiotherapy, but the majority should receive more invasive treatments, including calcaneal osteotomies or tendon debridement, depending on their particular presentation and pathology. This review examines the various different facets of posterior heel pain that must be dealt with and the most up-to-date treatments for the same.

 Video content accompanies this article at http://www.foot.theclinics.com.

The cavovarus foot is a complex deformity that can be treated using multiple surgical procedures, ranging from soft tissue surgery to triple arthrodesis. Among these options, anterior midfoot tarsectomy is a three-dimensional closed-wedge osteotomy, traditionally performed slowly and progressively in a blind fashion, and remaining a challenge for unexperimented surgeons with variable outcomes. As such, we investigated and discussed the use of patient-specific cutting guides (PSCGs) in computer-assisted anterior midfoot tarsectomy in terms of accuracy, reproducibility, and safety.

The aim of hindfoot fusions in the cavovarus foot is to establish a painless, plantigrade, balanced and stable foot. A comprehensive clinical and radiographic assessment enables the surgeon to fully understand the patient's deformity and plan a reliable surgical strategy for deformity correction. Pre-operative planning and intraoperative techniques are discussed.

Video content accompanies this article at http://www.foot.theclinics. com.

Cavovarus foot is a complex 3-dimensional deformity. Clinical history, physical examination, and comorbidity assessment are essential for preoperative evaluation. In severe cases, ankle or tibiotalocalcaneal arthrodesis can provide symptomatic relief and result in a plantigrade foot. This article emphasizes the importance of weight-bearing computed tomography for surgical planning and presents the authors' preferred technique for tibiotalocalcaneal, which includes a novel curved anterolateral incision, partial fibular onlay bridging graft, and patient-specific instrumentation for forefoot deformity correction. The tips and tricks aim to assist surgeons in better treating these challenging patients while optimizing preoperative planning.

Because of the good functional results and satisfactory implant survival achieved with modern models, total ankle replacement (TAR) has become a legitimate alternative to ankle fusion. However, alignment and balance are mandatory for implant survival. Satisfactory results can be achieved in patients with significant preoperative deformity if alignment and balance were obtained. If not, a staged procedure involving deformity correction and secondary TAR is possible. The authors describe the principal aspects of this concept and illustrate their current approach to TAR in cavovarus deformity.

Supramalleolar osteotomy enables correction of the ankle varus deformity and is associated with improvement of pain and function in the short term and long term. Despite these beneficial results, the amount of surgical correction is challenging to titrate and the procedure remains technically demanding. Most supramalleolar osteotomies are currently planned preoperatively on 2-dimensional weight-bearing radiographs and executed peroperatively using free-hand techniques. This article encompasses 3-dimensional planning and printing techniques based on weight-bearing computed tomography images and patient-specific instruments to correct ankle varus deformities.

In Charcot-Marie-Tooth (CMT) cavovarus surgery, a regimented approach is critical to create a plantigrade foot, restore hindfoot stability, and generate active ankle dorsiflexion. The preoperative motor examination is fundamental to the algorithm, as it is not only guides the initial surgical planning but is key in the decision making that occurs throughout the operation. Surgeons need to be comfortable with multiple techniques to achieve each surgical goal. There is no one operation that works for all patients with CMT. A plantigrade foot is the most important of the surgical goals as hindfoot stability and ankle dorsiflexion can be augmented with bracing.

A cavovarus foot is characterized by exacerbated medial longitudinal arch (cavus), hindfoot varus, plantar flexed first ray, forefoot pronation (apparent supination), forefoot adduction, and claw toe deformities. It can be broadly divided as flexible and rigid and further classified based on the neurological and non-neurological causes. Diabetes associated peripheral neuropathy complicates individual bony deformities associated with cavovarus foot with early callus which can breakdown to ulceration rapidly. Based on the disease progression in neurological and non-neurological causes of cavovarus feet in patients with diabetic neuropathy, 3 stages of the disease and its management is described.

The foot resembles a tripod. The 3 legs consist of (1) the tip of the heel, (2) the first metatarsal, and (3) the fifth metatarsal. This concept is useful to explain cavus or flat feet. When the tips of the tripod move closer, the arch becomes higher. The leg of the tripod that moves the most will determine the type of cavus feet, which can be hindfoot cavus, forefoot cavus, or first metatarsal cavus. Cavovarus foot denotes the presence of a three-dimensional deformity of the foot, but it is much more a descriptive feature than a diagnosis.

FOOT AND ANKLE CLINICS

RELATED SERIES

Orthopedic Clinics
Clinics in Sports Medicine
Physical Medicine and Rehabilitation Clinics

THE CLINICS ARE NOW AVAILABLE ONLINE!
Access your subscription at:
www.theclinics.com

Preface

Cavovarus Feet in 2023: Why We Should Look "Outside the Box"

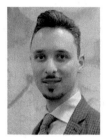

Alessio Bernasconi, MD, PhD, FEBOT
Editor

It was a great honor and privilege to serve as guest editor for this issue of *Foot and Ankle Clinics of North America* entitled "Innovative Approaches on Cavovarus Deformity: Thinking Outside of the Box."

When we say "cavovarus," we often simplify the description of a much more complex, three-dimensional foot shape, which requires all the possible attention in order to be correctly managed. The range of potential clinical scenarios related to the cavovarus foot is incredibly wide, going from milder forms with minor symptoms to painful and disabling conditions. Before looking at (and to better understand) what's "outside the box," we believe it's paramount to remind what's "inside" it! Especially for the youngest colleagues, we'd like to highlight the importance of what we already know in terms of anatomy and pathophysiology and what we already perform in terms of physical assessment, which in 2023 still retains an essential place in our practice. Understanding the complicated chain of events that leads to altering the normal anatomy and ultimately to the cavovarus drift is a challenge! Performing a correct clinical examination of the foot (pain location, reducibility, motor and sensory function in each anatomical plane, and so on) is still nowadays the starting point for every possible diagnostic and therapeutic pathway. This explains why you will see these concepts in the introduction section of a number of articles of this issue, which will likely help you get the greatest benefit from the advanced concepts explored and developed by our authors.

Every orthopedic surgeon dealing with cavovarus feet knows that it is often very difficult to correctly balance them and to reduce the overloading inherently related to their altered shape. We are still frequently unable to stop the progressive stiffening of soft tissue and joint degeneration, ending up with solutions that inevitably reduce the mobility of the foot and may limit the function and the gait of patients. We think

Foot Ankle Clin N Am 28 (2023) xv–xvi
https://doi.org/10.1016/j.fcl.2023.06.004
1083-7515/23/© 2023 Published by Elsevier Inc.

as emblematic all those correctible cavovarus in which twisting actually occurs at multiple levels (subtalar joint, Chopart joint, naviculocuneiform joints, and Lisfranc joint), but we usually proceed to realign only at the hindfoot (calcaneal osteotomy) and the forefoot (first metatarsal osteotomy), overall restoring a satisfactory foot tripod but de facto creating a sort of "Z" deformity. Also, there is still a lot of uncertainty around questions such as whether performing a calcaneal osteotomy when dealing with chronic lateral ankle instability really impacts clinical outcomes. These are simple examples of where the need to think "outside the box" comes from!

Most of the older and newer challenges related to cavovarus feet have been extensively discussed in this issue by world-renowned experts, who have kindly agreed to share their incredible experience in this field. Specifically, their management in specific populations (such as athletes, skeletally immature patients, patients diagnosed with diabetes or with neurologic conditions) has been deeply analyzed, providing tips that might be extremely useful to each one of us in daily clinics. The same applies to hindfoot and ankle arthrodeses, which must remain in the armamentarium of the surgeon for treating stiff degenerated joints, but which are still characterized by a non-negligible rate of failure. Furthermore, the role of cone-beam weight-bearing computed tomography in the diagnostic pathway of cavovarus-related conditions, as a way to define the true CORA (Centre of Rotation and Angulation) or CORAs of the deformity, plan correction with greater accuracy, and, in turn, improve outcomes, has been summarized. Last, but certainly not least, the state-of-the-art about new techniques (such as minimally invasive procedures, last-generation total ankle replacement, or supramalleolar and midfoot osteotomies guided by patient-specific instrumentation) has been defined, highlighting their huge potential in the setting of cavovarus feet correction but also discussing knowledge gaps still awaiting to be covered.

To conclude, let me warmly thank the Editor-in-Chief of *Foot and Ankle Clinics of North America*, Cesar de Cesar Netto, for his friendship, for being such an inspirational colleague, for trusting us with the management of this issue, and for helping me gather such an incredible international faculty. I'd also like to sincerely thank every single author who agreed to contribute to this issue and dedicate part of their precious time to its creation. Without them, the publication of this issue would not have been possible.

And now, just click on the next link (if you are online) or please turn the page (if you have it in your hands), dive deep, and enjoy the reading!

Alessio Bernasconi, MD, PhD, FEBOT
Trauma and Orthopaedic Unit
Department of Public Health
University Federico II of Naples
Via Pansini 5
Naples 80131, Italy

E-mail address:
alebernas@gmail.com

The Role Of Minimally Invasive Osteotomies In Cavovarus Foot Reconstruction: Detailed Technique And Evidence For Procedures

Razi Zaidi, BSc (Hons), MD, FRCS (Tr & Orth),
Thomas Lorchan Lewis, BSc (Hons), MBChB (Hons), MFSTEd, FRCS (Tr & Orth),
Robbie Ray, MB, ChB, ChM (T&O), FRCSed(Tr & Orth), FEBOT*

KEYWORDS

- Calcaneal osteotomy • Metatarsal osteotomy • Minimally invasive surgery
- Percutaneous surgery • Cavovarus deformity

KEY POINTS

- Surgical management of cavovarus foot reconstruction is an individualized combination of surgical procedures designed to correct deformity.
- Minimally invasive procedures using high-torque low-speed burr can facilitate large deformity correction without extensive soft tissue stripping.

INTRODUCTION

A cavus foot is defined as a high-arched foot that fails to flatten on weight-bearing. Causes are numerous and can be either congenital or acquired, affecting both children and adults. People with cavus foot may experience pain, instability, and difficulty with balance and walking, which can significantly influence their quality of life.

Studies have reported the prevalence of cavus foot to be between 0% and 10% of the general population. However, the incidence is higher in certain populations, such as those with neurological conditions such as Charcot-Marie-Tooth disease or cerebral palsy. In these populations, the incidence can be as high as 80%.

The etiology of cavus foot is multifactorial and can result from various underlying conditions, including neurological disorders such as Charcot-Marie-Tooth disease, spinal cord injuries, and cerebral palsy, as well as musculoskeletal conditions such

King's Foot and Ankle Unit, King's College Hospital NHS Foundation Trust, London SE5 9RS, UK
* Corresponding author.
E-mail address: robbie.ray2@nhs.net

Foot Ankle Clin N Am 28 (2023) 709–718
https://doi.org/10.1016/j.fcl.2023.05.002
1083-7515/23/© 2023 Elsevier Inc. All rights reserved.

foot.theclinics.com

as clubfoot, poliomyelitis, and trauma. These conditions lead to muscular imbalances between the intrinsic and extrinsic musculatures that result in the deformity.

Often cavus feet present a diagnostic and therapeutic challenge for foot and ankle surgeons. Deformity is translational and rotational deformity in the sagittal, axial, and coronal planes, occurring at multiple levels.[1]

Traditional techniques to correct cavus deformity have often been in the form of open surgery. The current study presents minimally invasive surgical techniques for the management of cavus foot.

INDICATIONS AND CONTRAINDICATIONS

Surgery for cavus foot is indicated when conservative treatment options, such as orthotics and physiotherapy, have been unsuccessful in improving symptoms and function.[2] Indications for surgery may include severe foot pain, instability, and difficulty with walking and balance.[3] The goal of surgery is to improve foot function and mobility by correcting deformity and giving the patient a plantigrade, stable, painless foot. Specific type of surgery depends on the underlying deformity. Common procedures would include osteotomies in order to correct deformity supplemented with soft tissue procedures. Fusion operations maybe indicated in rigid deformities.

PATIENT HISTORY/PHYSICAL EXAMINATION

History and examination are important tenants of any management process. History should focus on the exact source of pain and duration. Instability may also be a factor that needs to be uncovered. It is also important to ascertain what treatment the patient has had and what the expectations and hopes are for any future management. Family history is also important in order to focus on the presence of hereditary neurological conditions such as Charcot-Marie-Tooth (CMT).

The cavus foot has reduced forefoot and subtalar movement, reducing the ability to absorb impact at initial contact. Callosities result at the lateral heel base and head fifth met and first met head, often hallux sesamoiditis. Patients may also complain fatigability. Internal torque may produce ankle and subtalar inversion sprains/instability. Patients may also have suffered metatarsal stress fractures or present with peroneal tendon pathologic condition.

Clinical examination should be started by observing the gait for foot drop. General inspection may show muscle wasting and callosities under areas of pressure. Range of motion in every joint should be examined and determine whether it is stiff or rigid. Lower limb neurology should also be documented. The gastrocnemius may also be tight and a Silfverskiold test will show this. This is important because the gastrocnemius recession may be added to the surgery to get the foot plantigrade. The Coleman block test is probably the most known test done in this condition.[4] A positive Coleman block sign implies that the hindfoot varus is due to the plantarflexed first ray and that the hindfoot is flexible.

In summary, after clinical evaluation, we should know whether the patients' deformities are rigid or flexible. We should also have an idea as to the neurological status.

IMAGING STUDIES

Imaging is important for surgical decision-making. Ideally, weight-bearing, computed tomography (CT) will demonstrate the deformities of interest and any joint degenerative pathologic condition. This mode of imaging has gained popularity in recent years.[5,6]

In the absence of weight-bearing, CT, all patients should have weight-bearing images of the foot and ankle. An anterior posterior (AP) view may show a decreased talo—first metatarsal angle. On the lateral view, an increased Meary angle, decreased talar declination, increased calcaneal pitch (Pitch) angle may be seen. Imaging of the ankle shows if arthritis or deformity exists.

PREOPERATIVE PLANNING AND PREPARATION

The set up for minimally invasive surgery (MIS) procedures is of the utmost importance in order to improve the flow and efficiency of the procedure. The main aims of the setup are as follows.

- The surgeon should be well positioned to use the burr with their dominant hand.
- There must be adequate space and planning to use an image intensifier/mini c-arm throughout the procedure without risking sterility or the comfort of the surgeon.
- The nurse or surgical technician should be positioned so that they are available to pass instruments without impeding the surgeon or image intensifier.

For calcaneal osteotomy, the ideal position is for the leg to be in a lateral position. The senior author prefers "the floppy lateral" position, which allows for knee flexion to give a good lateral position and for knee extension and hip external rotation to give a good AP position for radiographs and medial procedures (**Fig. 1**).

The authors do not recommend the use of supine position, and a sandbag as a true lateral of the calcaneus is challenging in this position and inadvertent straying of the burr toward the subtalar joint is more likely in this position.

Right-handed surgeons should always position themselves behind the patient for calcaneal osteotomy. This allows for full access to the calcaneus by moving between the side of the patient and the foot of the bed and puts their dominant hand in a relaxed position to operate and complete the osteotomy using a supinatory movement. For calcaneal osteotomy, the image intensifier or mini c-arm should be brought in from the opposite side of the patient from the surgeon so as not to impede access to the patient's foot.

Another important aspect of imaging positioning is that the imaging machine should be arranged so that the plate or drum is used as a table on which the heel rests (image). It is our preference to use a mini c-arm over a large image intensifier. The other

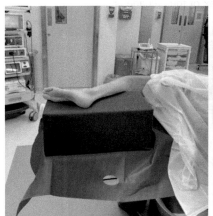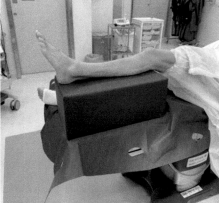

Fig. 1. The patient positioning and ease of access for both AP and lateral views.

important factor to consider is that many orthopedic procedures are performed in theaters with a laminar flow perspex box, and because the commonly performed procedure being lower limb arthroplasty, the bed is generally positioned with the feet at the edge of this box. If this is the case, the perspex box can impede access for the imaging machine especially if it is a larger machine and due care must be taken to position the patient deeper into the laminar flow perspex box before beginning the procedure.

The nurse or surgical technician should be positioned such that they are not in the way of the surgeon and able to assist throughout the procedure. As such, for a right-handed surgeon, we position the nurse to the left of the patient behind the surgeon. From this position, the assistant has ample space to open their trays and have their equipment ready. The console for the MIS system and power instruments should be set up at the patient's right hip out of the operating field. This allows for the cables from the MIS console and drills to come across the bed and remain sterile throughout the procedure (**Fig. 2**).

SURGICAL TECHNIQUE
Surgical Technique: MIS Calcaneal Osteotomy

The procedure is typically performed under general anesthesia and lower limb nerve blockade. A tourniquet is routinely used for this procedure. Once the patient is appropriately positioned, the osteotomy is marked out on the skin using a stout k wire and a marking pen. The senior author finds that the k wires used for the 7-mm calcaneal screws is ideal for this. An initial oblique line is marked in the plane of the osteotomy. This should be from dorsal proximal to plantar distal exiting proximal to the plantar fascia insertion so that the shift is not hindered by tightness in this structure. A second perpendicular line is drawn at the midpoint of the calcaneus, which gives the skin incision point and also a guide for the screws, which can be inserted slightly above and below parallel to this line (**Fig. 3**).

The wire is then inserted subcutaneously in line with the osteotomy line and checked on x-ray (**Fig. 4**).

The idea is that by burring against the posterior aspect of the wire, the plane of the osteotomy can be kept in check and the risk of anterior translation of the osteotomy risking the subtalar joint can be reduced.[7]

A 3/30 burr is used for calcaneal osteotomy. The 3-mm thickness allows for adequate bone removal to allow for a good shift while the 30-mm length allows for adequate depth to easily reach the far cortex of the calcaneus.

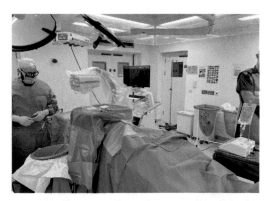

Fig. 2. Operating room setup demonstrating relevant positioning of instruments and mini c-arm.

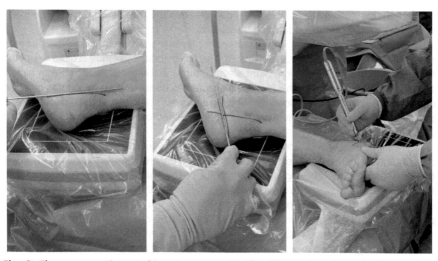

Fig. 3. The preoperative marking to accurately identify the location of the calcaneal osteotomy.

The senior surgeon's technique involves making a 3 to 5-mm skin incision at the bisection of the skin markings and using an artery clamp to clear soft tissues down to bone. A periosteal elevator is then used to clear soft tissues and periosteum dorsal and plantar. The burr is then inserted around an open artery clamp to protect the sural nerve and inserted bicortical to the far cortex. This ensures the burr is set at an adequate length to complex the osteotomy. The near cortices and dorsal and plantar cortices are then cut using a combination of supinatory wrist movement and gentle pushing of the burr to ensure the arc included all plantar cortices. To ensure comfortable completion, the moves from the side of the bed to the foot of the bed for the dorsal and plantar halves of the cuts to avoid a back hand technique. Once the near dorsal and plantar cortices are completed, the far cortex is completed using the channel made as a guide. The wire is kept in place throughout to act as a guide also. For beginners, care must be taken not to damage the posteromedial structures on the far side of the osteotomy. Straying into these structures leads to uncontrolled toe flexion, and if this is seen, the burr must be drawn back to avoid iatrogenic injury.

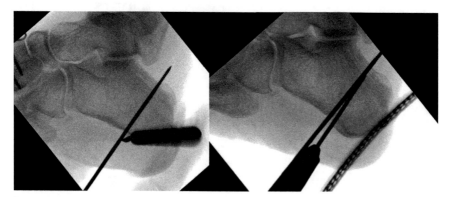

Fig. 4. Intraoperative imaging demonstrating a percutaneous calcaneal osteotomy using a k-wire to guide the burr.

Once the osteotomy is completed, it can be seen that the osteotomy will be freely mobile with easy medial and lateral translation.

To gain a good correction, the senior author finds that a percutaneous medial incision at the osteotomy is safe and effective. The floppy lateral position is used to put the leg in an AP position. Passing a blunt elevator through the osteotomy, a 3-mm nick in the skin is made medially. This is blunt dissected to bone, and an elevator is inserted into the distal body of the calcaneus. The leg is moved back into a lateral position, and the elevator is fulcrummed against the table to allow for maximal lateral translation (**Fig. 5**).

The patient is now well positioned for wire and screw insertion. Using the marking perpendicular to the osteotomy as a guide, 2 wires are inserted above and below this line. As we are valgising, the entry point of the wires should be just medial to the midline of the calcaneus aiming slightly lateral distally. Once position in the proximal fragment is confirmed, elevation of the hand will put a further valgus force on the proximal fragment and the wires can be driven into the calcaneal body. At this point, an axial calcaneal view is necessary. This is easily achieved with a mini c-arm utilizing a modified magneto technique.[8] The foot is kept in the lateral position and dorsiflexed and the mini c-arm is turned 90° with the heel on the plate, which gives an excellent view of the calcaneus, and wires can be adjusted as necessary. Wires are then over-drilled and compression screws are inserted (**Fig. 6**).

Surgical Technique: MIS First MT Basal Osteotomy

To perform the basal osteotomy, the AP position of the floppy lateral is used. The first tarsometatarsal joint (TMT) is marked under x-ray and a 3-mm medial incision is made 1 cm distal to the TMT joint. An artery clip is used to spread soft tissues and a periosteal elevator is used to clear dorsal and plantar soft tissues (**Fig. 7**).

A 2/20 mm burr is used to make the initial osteotomy. If the burr system for the calcaneal osteotomy uses a 3/20 burr rather than a 3/30 mm burr, then the same burr can be used here. A 3/30 burr, however, is too long to give adequate control when making a basal osteotomy of the first metatarsal. The osteotomy is a dorsal closing wedge aiming to elevate the first ray. The cortices to be cut are the dorsal, medial, and lateral (**Fig. 8**).

The senior author aims to keep the plantar medial cortex and remove the plantar lateral corner because this is the thickest bone in the metatarsal, and taking this

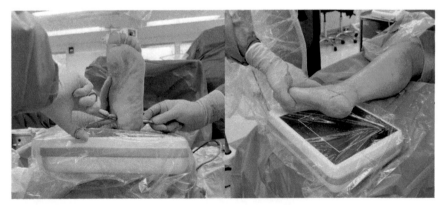

Fig. 5. Medial percutaneous access for elevator to be inserted to perform the reduction maneuver to achieve lateral translation, which is confirmed on imaging.

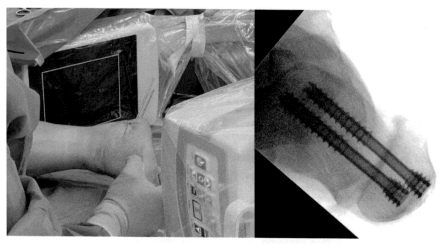

Fig. 6. The calcaneal osteotomy is held with k-wires and stabilized with 2 cannulated screws.

bone allows for gentle closure of the osteotomy with cracking the plantar cortex and completing the osteotomy, which can make the osteotomy unstable. The senior author always makes the osteotomy from dorsal distal to plantar proximal. This allows for the screw to be inserted from proximal to distal closing the osteotomy and not risking encroachment to the first TMT joint. The surgeon stands on the left of the patient for a left foot or between the legs for the right foot and completes the osteotomy with a supinatory action. If more bone needs to be taken, the burr can be swept along the same path again, or for very big corrections, a wedge burr can be used to increase the wedge. It should be noted that the more bone that is removed, the more shortening occurs, and the senior author finds that usually a few passes of the 2/20 shannon burr suffices. The osteotomy should then close with gentle finger pressure. A wire is then inserted from dorso medial at the TMT joint aiming distal lateral across the osteotomy and a 4-mm screw is used to fix the osteotomy (**Fig. 9**).

Ideally, a compression screw should be used but the senior author generally uses an MIS screw as the bevelled head reduces the risk of screw prominence. If the osteotomy is inadvertently completed, care should be taken to hold the first MT in an adequately dorsiflexed position and use the wire and screw to maintain this position. Once fixed, this osteotomy should also be quite stable because it is a closing wedge.

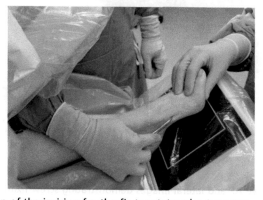

Fig. 7. The location of the incision for the first metatarsal osteotomy.

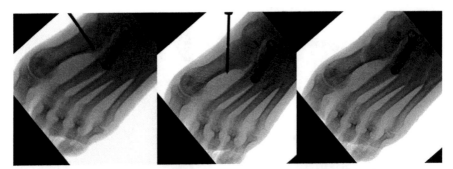

Fig. 8. Intraoperative images demonstrating the proximal first metatarsal osteotomy.

The wounds are carefully inspected for any sign of skin thermal damage in which case the skin edges are excised to reduce the risk of postoperative wound problems. The incisions are closed with 4-0 monocryl subcuticular sutures. The foot is wrapped with gauze, webril cotton dressing, and a plaster backslab.

POSTOPERATIVE MANAGEMENT

Minimally invasive calcaneal and first metatarsal dorsiflexion osteotomies can be performed on an outpatient basis although patients have to mobilize with non–weight-bearing so may need admission for physiotherapy. Patients are counseled regarding the importance of elevating the foot in the first 2 weeks following surgery to reduce swelling and the risk of wound problems. At 2 weeks postop, patients are allowed to transition to a walking boot or walking cast as pain allows and are encouraged to gradually increase walking as tolerated. Patients start removing the boot after 6 weeks, and complete recovery can take 6 months or longer depending on additional procedures (**Fig. 10**).

OUTCOMES

The current study presents minimal invasive techniques in the management of cavus foot deformities. Research in this area has been quite minimal and limited to small case-series.

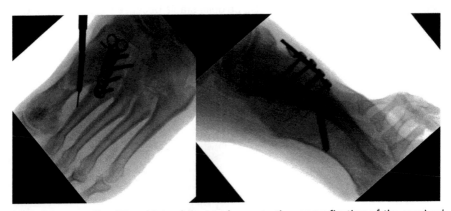

Fig. 9. Intraoperative AP and lateral images demonstrating screw fixation of the proximal first metatarsal osteotomy.

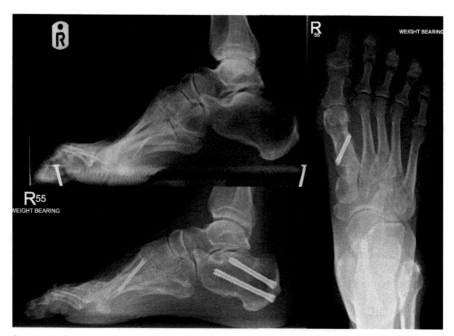

Fig. 10. Radiographs demonstrating the preoperative and postoperative correction that can be achieved with percutaneous cavus foot reconstruction.

A group from Brazil presented their results of 20 cavus corrections.[9] They were corrected using first metatarsal osteotomy and calcaneal osteotomy. They demonstrated good, hindfoot, correction. All the metatarsal osteotomies healed. They had no wound complications. However, there was a 60% sural nerve injury rate. Other studies comparing with minimally invasive calcaneal osteotomies to open have shown it to be safe.[10,11] The Oxford group found a similar amount of shift achievable with both open and minimally invasive methods. Cadaveric studies show that minimally invasive methods have a low risk of nerve injury.[12] Use of radiographic assistance for MIS calcaneal osteotomies has also been shown to have significant improvements in postoperative radiographic and functional outcomes from baseline to 6 months postoperatively, demonstrating its use as a safe and effective means of treating hindfoot malalignment.[13]

Complications

Complications following MIS calcaneal osteotomies are generally low. A comparative study of open versus percutaneous osteotomies found higher wound healing rates in the open cohort as well as a prolonged length of stay.[14]

SUMMARY

Percutaneous correction of cavus foot deformity can be achieved with satisfactory correction of foot anatomy and biomechanics. Surgical management of cavovarus foot reconstruction is an individualized combination of surgical procedures designed to correct deformity. Minimally invasive procedures using high-torque low-speed burr can facilitate large deformity correction without extensive soft tissue stripping. However, there is a lack of methodologically robust evidence to support this procedure at present and further research, particularly, focusing on long-term clinical outcomes and follow-up is required.

DISCLOSURE

R. Ray reports fees from Marquadt outside the scope of this article. None of the other authors has any conflicts of interest.

REFERENCES

1. Kaplan JRM, Aiyer A, Cerrato RA, et al. Operative treatment of the cavovarus foot. Foot Ankle Int 2018;39(11):1370–82.
2. Burns J, Landorf KB, Ryan MM, et al. Interventions for the prevention and treatment of pes cavus. Cochrane Database Syst Rev 2007;2007(4):CD006154.
3. Akoh CC, Phisitkul P. Clinical examination and radiographic assessment of the cavus foot. Foot Ankle Clin 2019;24(2):183–93.
4. Coleman SS, Chesnut WJ. A simple test for hindfoot flexibility in the cavovarus foot. Clin Orthop Relat Res 1977;(123):60–2.
5. Kvarda P, Krähenbühl N, Susdorf R, et al. High reliability for semiautomated 3D measurements based on weightbearing CT scans. Foot Ankle Int 2022; 43(1):91–5.
6. Pfeffer GB, Michalski M, Nelson T, et al. Extensor tendon transfers for treatment of foot drop in charcot-marie-tooth disease: a biomechanical evaluation. Foot Ankle Int 2020;41(4):449–56.
7. Lee M, Guyton GP, Zahoor T, et al. Minimally invasive calcaneal displacement osteotomy site using a reference kirschner wire: a technique tip. J Foot Ankle Surg 2016;55(5):1121–6.
8. Newman ET, Kelly BA, Rodriguez EK. The "magneto view": a simple method for obtaining intraoperative axial radiographs of the calcaneus. The Orthopaedic Journal at Harvard Medical School 2015;16:116–20.
9. Astolfi RS, de Vasconcelos Coelho JV, Ribeiro HCT, et al. Cavus foot correction using a full percutaneous procedure: a case series. Int J Environ Res Publ Health 2021;18(19). https://doi.org/10.3390/ijerph181910089.
10. Kendal AR, Khalid A, Ball T, et al. Complications of minimally invasive calcaneal osteotomy versus open osteotomy. Foot Ankle Int 2015;36(6):685–90.
11. Coleman MM, Abousayed MM, Thompson JM, et al. Risk factors for complications associated with minimally invasive medial displacement calcaneal osteotomy. Foot Ankle Int 2020;42(2):121–31.
12. Durston A, Bahoo R, Kadambande S, et al. Minimally invasive calcaneal osteotomy: does the shannon burr endanger the neurovascular structures? A cadaveric study. J Foot Ankle Surg 2015;54(6):1062–6.
13. Veljkovic A, Symes M, Younger A, et al. Neurovascular and clinical outcomes of the percutaneous endoscopically assisted calcaneal osteotomy (PECO) technique to correct hindfoot malalignment. Foot Ankle Int 2019;40(2):178–84.
14. Gutteck N, Zeh A, Wohlrab D, et al. Comparative results of percutaneous calcaneal osteotomy in correction of hindfoot deformities. Foot Ankle Int 2019;40(3): 276–81.

Cavovarus Deformity: Why Weight-Bearing Computed Tomography Should Be a First-Line Imaging Modality

François Lintz, MD, MSc, FEBOT[a],*, Alessio Bernasconi, MD, PhD, FEBOT[b]

KEYWORDS

- Cavovarus • Weight-bearing CT • WBCT • Foot • Deformity • Three-dimensional

KEY POINTS

- Cavovarus patients present with complex three-dimensional (3D) deformities responsible for mild to severe functional impairment: 3D weight-bearing assessment is therefore paramount to their improved understanding.
- The traditional 2D radiographs—computed tomography sequence, are time-consuming, heavy in terms of radiations, and present with unavoidable biases related to projections, superimposition (especially in cavovarus), and the absence of weight bearing.
- Modern visualization tools such as distance mapping and automatic measurements on images from cone-beam weight-bearing computed tomography provide new information and faster processing times.
- The ultimate goal is to improve the accuracy of surgical planning and clinical outcome for complex deformities such as cavovarus feet.

INTRODUCTION

Cavovarus deformity is defined as a three-dimensional (3D) alteration of the physiologic foot shape involving simultaneously the hindfoot, the midfoot, and the forefoot.[1] The ankle is often involved as well, the leg being externally rotated relative to the talar dome. In this sense, it is clear that 3D weight-bearing imaging is a great added value compared with two-dimensional (2D) or non-weight-bearing conventional imaging. Although multiple causes can be identified, cavovarus feet may be considered either idiopathic or secondary (to central or peripheral neurologic conditions, clubfoot, polio, rheumatological diseases or deformities from previous fractures).[2,3] Apart from clearly pathologic conditions, a specific entity dubbed "subtle cavovarus" was described by Manoli and Graham. This "underpronator" foot was defined as an idiopathic, familial,

[a] Ramsay Santé Clinique de l'Union, Centre de Chirurgie de la Cheville et du Pied, Saint Jean, France; [b] Department of Public Health, Orthopaedic and Traumatology Unit, University Federico II of Naples, Naples, Italy
* Corresponding author.
E-mail address: dr.f.lintz@gmail.com

Foot Ankle Clin N Am 28 (2023) 719–728
https://doi.org/10.1016/j.fcl.2023.05.001
1083-7515/23/© 2023 Elsevier Inc. All rights reserved.

and not really genetically determined form of cavovarus foot.[4] Interestingly, the investigators stated that the subtle cavovarus may also be secondary to neurologic conditions, which would not be entirely in agreement with the concept of "idiopathic" and has never been really clarified.[4] From a structural standpoint, in their paper, the investigators also discussed the chain of events, which leads to the final cavovarus shape. They acknowledged the difference between a forefoot-driven and a hindfoot-driven cavovarus foot, although they stated that subtle cavovarus was generally related to the first form. At the beginning, a hyper-plantarflexion of the first ray (which is without a clear cause, the main hypothesis being the "peroneal overdrive" hyperactivity of the peroneus longus which attaches to the plantar aspect of the first metatarsal) leads to the pronation of the forefoot. This generates a paradoxical supination as soon as it leads to the ground as an adaptation of the forefoot to a flat surface (**Fig. 1**). This supination results in a progressive supination (varization) of the hindfoot, which adapts to the forefoot rotation. This brings to a progressive lack of eversion at the subtalar joint (in a sort of locked inversion). If the deforming forces keep acting, a gradual stiffening of the deformity is generally observed (from flexible, to stiff, to rigid). At the same time, a progressive tightening of the triceps surae and Achilles tendon often occurs, also as a result of the plantarflexion of the first ray which brings the head of the first metatarsal lower than the heel weight-bearing point. Biomechanically, this further weakens the tibialis anterior action which in turn reduces its antagonist effect against the peroneus longus, therefore feeding the "peroneal overdrive" mentioned above.[4] In this context and aware of such pathophysiology, a thorough physical examination is keystone to understand which joints and tendons are involved in this pathologic process and to distinguish between a flexible and a rigid deformity. In our mind, however, performing technological tools become the clinical input will always be paramount in this setting.

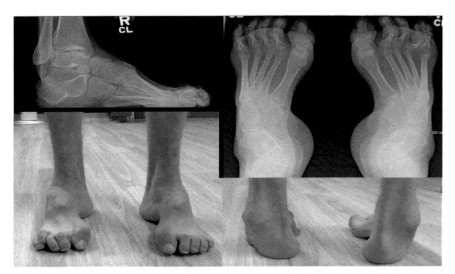

Fig. 1. Example of a 22-year-old gentleman diagnosed with Charcot–Marie–Tooth and presenting with symptomatic bilateral cavovarus deformity. In a lateral foot radiograph (*top left image*), the ankle joint appears externally rotated and becoming similar to an anteroposterior view. In dorsoplantar feet radiographs (*top right image*), the significant supination of the midfoot may be appreciated with the talonavicular joint almost being lateral to the calcaneocuboid joint. The clinical presentation has been showed in the bottom images, with both feet observed during stance from the front (*bottom left image*) and the back (*bottom right image*).

First-line imaging is traditionally based on standing radiographs with multiple projections (ie, dorsoplantar and lateral view of both feet, anteroposterior view of both ankles, hindfoot alignment view of both hindfeet). These are mainly used to get an overview, as the only weight-bearing imaging available until a decade ago, of the foot and ankle alignment through angles and axes. To evaluate the status of joints, a computed tomography (CT) may be requested, exposing the patient to a higher dose of radiations (as compared with radiographs) and loosing all the alignment information. The following paragraphs will be dedicated to explain why cone-beam weight-bearing CT (WBCT) overcomes these limitations and should represent the first-line imaging in the assessment of 3D deformities such as cavovarus feet.

RADIOGRAPHS AND CONVENTIONAL COMPUTED TOMOGRAPHY

Biases related to radiographs in foot and ankle surgery have been widely discussed in literature.[5–7] The limitations of 2D imaging should be borne in mind especially in the study of 3D complex deformities as in the case of cavovarus feet.

First, looking at a traditional dorsoplantar and lateral radiograph of a cavovarus foot, it is difficult is to distinguish the contour of midfoot bones. Although such bones (especially the three cuneiforms and the cuboid with their medial, lateral, proximal, and distal contours) are already slightly superimposed in normal feet (which often brings the clinician to request a specific oblique dorsoplantar view with the beam oriented from dorsolateral to plantar-medial), they appear even more overlapped than usual in cavovarus deformities due to the supination of the midfoot (see **Fig. 1**). Even the talonavicular joint might be almost completely dorsal to the calcaneocuboid joint, making interpretation hard at the Chopart joint as well.

Second, achieving a correct rotation of the foot during the acquisition of the image is paramount to get a standardized and reproducible result (ie, for pretreatment and posttreatment comparison or to assess interindividual differences in a definite cohort of patients). There is good consensus in literature to represent the longitudinal axis of the foot as the long axis of the second metatarsal bone. This is confirmed by investigators such as Saltzman and El-Khoury (which introduced the homonymous view to assess hindfoot alignment) or Reilingh (who introduced the long axial view); they all recommended aligning the foot along the axis of the second metatarsal.[8,9] In cavovarus deformities, aligning the foot in a "standardized" fashion might be challenging. The varus and supination of the hindfoot coupled with the adduction and supination of the forefoot create a bean-shape effect, which means that the hindfoot would appear completely rotated in standard hindfoot views (**Fig. 2**). This might wrongly lead the technician to put the foot straight on the ground and take the image positioning the source from the back, which would likely false any kind of measurement and strongly limit its reproducibility. Among others, a cadaveric study by Baverel and colleagues has mathematically confirmed that rotating the foot affects the accuracy of hindfoot alignment measurements.[5]

The third type of bias (somehow similar to the second one) is the variability of technical operations, which in part regards the settings of the radiographic source and in part the orientation of the beam. As the definition of cavovarus foot actually includes a wide range of possible shapes (ie, the equinus could be less or more accentuated with difficulty to engage the heel to the ground or high-arches could be predominant as compared with the varus heel, or the whole foot could be entirely supinated with the lateral aspect of the midfoot becoming the weight-bearing part of the structure, and so on), it is not possible at the moment to provide guidelines to align "correctly" the source of radiations to take images. If these elements might only partially influence

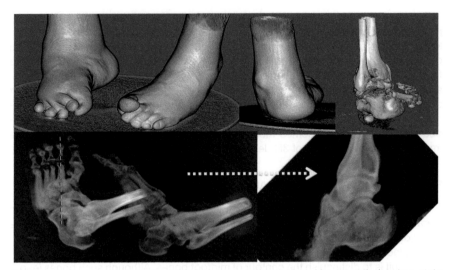

Fig. 2. Soft-tissue rendering (*top left and top central image*) and bony rendering (*top right image*) for weight-bearing images of a patient diagnosed with bilateral cavovarus foot. In the bottom left image, an example of how the foot could be aligned along the axis of the second metatarsal. By rotating this image and looking at the foot from the back (to obtain a Saltzman view), the observer would visualize a sort of lateral view of the hindfoot (*bottom right image*), making measurements likely biased by the important rotation of the whole anatomical area.

measurements taken on subtle cavovarus feet, they certainly need to be taken into account for severely deformed feet.

Because of these limitations and of the limited contrast resolution inherently related to radiographs, clinicians have traditionally relied on CT scans to assess the true bone morphology and to evaluate the relationship between bones at the joint interface. The absence of gravity means that joint spaces seen through standard CT do not reflect what really happens during stance; therefore, variable interpretation has to be undertaken by physicians in translating what's been seen on CT and radiographs and plan correctly any potential surgery.

WEIGHT-BEARING COMPUTED TOMOGRAPHY IN CAVOVARUS FEET

Since the first publications approximately a decade ago reporting the use of WBCT in foot and ankle surgery, there has been an increasing interest toward this innovative imaging modality due to the possibility to acquire images in an upright position and with a reduced dose of radiations (cone beam technology).[10,11] With regard to cavovarus feet, a few papers have recently been published dealing with the role of WBCT in the management of these conditions. In 2020, Bernasconi and colleagues investigated the reliability of 3D semiautomatic measurements (defined semiautomatic as the observer has to select by hand precise landmarks based on which a dedicated software then runs the calculation) such as the Foot and Ankle Offset, the Calcaneal Offset, and the Hindfoot Alignment Angle in the assessment of hindfoot alignment in pes cavovarus.[12] The investigators found an excellent intraobserver and interobserver agreement for such measurements and also demonstrated that etiology (neurologic or non-neurologic), severity of deformity, and level of seniority of the observer did not influence their reliability.[12] The following year, the same investigators compared angular measurements and distances performed on idiopathic cavovarus feet with those taken on Charcot–Marie–Tooth (CMT).[13] Their preliminary findings suggested that CMT feet suffered from increased forefoot supination and more severe hindfoot malalignment as compared with idiopathic forms.[13] In another study by An and colleagues, WBCT images from 27 CMT feet and 20 healthy controls were compared.[14] The investigators demonstrated that a significant axial plane adduction and coronal plane rotation occurred at the talonavicular joint in CMT patients, concluding that the soft tissue release at this level might play a crucial role in the surgical correction of CMT feet.[14]

How to Assess Bones: Automatic Measurements for Angles and Axes

Automatic measurements have been recently proposed in the foot and ankle field as an attempt to obtain a number of measurements (axes and angles) in an accurate way but dramatically reducing the amount of time needed to calculate them. Richter and colleagues have analyzed 500 bilateral WBCT scans on which five measurements (including the hindfoot angle) had been calculated both by hand and semiautomatically.[15] They demonstrated a 73% reduction in terms of time spent to obtain angles (12 seconds vs 44 seconds), although they also found significant differences in measurements obtained by hand and semiautomatically and concluding that their validity was still to be demonstrated.[15] For what concerns cavovarus feet, a similar analysis was carried out by Sangoi and colleagues by comparing 16 CMT cavovarus feet with 16 normal feet.[16] In their study, six measurements were performed both manually on 2D slices and using a specialized software. Interestingly, although no significant bias was identified in normal feet (for which measurements obtained through the two methods were comparable), the investigators identified a tendency to overestimate the sagittal deformity (fixed bias 7.31° for Méary angle, 2.39° for calcaneal pitch) and underestimate the axial deformity (fixed bias 10.61° for axial talar−first metatarsal angle) for the automatic measurements.[16] In this last case, a proportional bias was also found indicating greater discrepancy with increasing adduction. The investigators hypothesized that such discrepancy could be explained by the rotational deformity seen in cavovarus feet, which could not be easily evaluated on 2D images.[16] Bearing these studies in mind, we deem it worth to remind that the current gold standard for the assessment of angles and axes in foot and ankle has been represented so far by by-hand measurements performed on radiographic images, which are nowadays considered "validated," as in multiple studies different observers have been finding similar results. However, if we assume that the rotational deformity, as just mentioned, is not easy to assess on radiograph, it is just possible that all the observers repeatedly perform the same error during measurements producing a bias. There are chances that this systematic error has never come up as no other imaging method was available in the past which could potentially overcome such limit and give back results that are closer to true angles. In other words, 2D images as gold standard probably inherently result in a standard error. Of course, this hypothesis will need to be confirmed or disproved by future robust studies on the topic.

Interestingly, in a study led by Michalski and colleagues, the osteology of CMT patients has also been investigated. The investigators found significant differences at the navicular tuberosity, medial talar head, sustentaculum tali, and anterior process of the calcaneus in CMT patients as compared with normal feet.[17] Although it must be acknowledged that the difference in bony structure could also theoretically be analyzed using non-weight-bearing imaging, we believe that the possibility to obtain the information about angles, axes, and bone morphology at once through WBCT represent a precious added value of such technology and may allow the clinician to obtain an accurate and quick evaluation of complex deformities in daily clinical practice.

How to Assess Joints: Distance Mapping

The assessment of the interaction of bones at joints can only be correctly performed on standing images. Before WBCT, this has routinely been done using radiographs and evaluating the narrowing or opening of joint spaces along with the congruence of the articular surfaces. At the time when this article is written, Kellgren–Lawrence (KL) classification represents the most common system used in clinical practice around the world to estimate the degree of degeneration (narrowing associated to osteophytes, bony sclerosis, and cysts) of a joint. To summarize, each osteoarthritic joint can be assigned a grade from 0 to 4 with Grade 0 signifying no presence of osteoarthrosis and Grade 4 signifying severe degeneration. The KL system has been widely used for major lower limb joints (hip and knees), but only few studies have assessed its reliability in foot and ankle joints. In a study by Vier and colleagues, where the investigators investigated the interobserver agreement of KL system on the subtalar joint, an overall fair reliability among reviewers (kappa = 0.26) was found.[18] In another study by Mayich and colleagues, the use of KL to assess the radiographic progression of osteoarthritis in the peritalar joints following total ankle replacement was evaluated.[19] Also in this case, the interrater reliability of KL was only moderate (kappa at 0.37 and 0.46 for the subtalar and talonavicular joint, respectively), bringing the investigators to state that such system was not a reliable tool for these patients.[19] What is maybe even more important is that, regardless of foot and ankle joints, it is widely known that a poor correlation exists between a radiographic assessment of a joint and the clinical status of a patient, that is, it is not possible to affirm that a patient with osteoarthritis of the ankle classified as KL 2 has more severe symptoms than another patient with an ankle osteoarthritis KL 3. This leads to the conclusion that joints should be assessed using different systems with a higher correlation with the clinical scenario.

In this context, distance mapping (DM) was introduced in the foot and ankle field by Siegler in 2018 as a tool to analyze the joint interaction at the foot and ankle.[20] In practical terms, the DM algorithm (run through dedicated software) allows to compute the distance distribution between two opposing articular surfaces, which is an indirect measure of the pressures exerted in a certain part of the joint. Although it should be emphasized that a map of distances does not necessarily reflect a map of pressures, some published works such as the one from Corazza and colleagues [21] seem to suggest that these two parameters may correspond, which obviously needs confirmation by further studies. It is clear that these algorithms require 3D imaging to be run and that the application of the force of gravity (like in WBCT) is necessary to study each joint in a configuration, which is similar as much as possible to the physiologic one.

Although a few studies have been published where DM was used to evaluate the joint status in acquired flatfoot,[22–24] to the best of our knowledge its value in cavovarus feet has been investigated only in one study by Lintz and colleagues.[25] In their comparative study, the investigators assessed the ankle, subtalar, talonavicular, naviculocuneiform, and tarsometatarsal joints of 10 cases and 10 controls, producing distance maps on images from WBCT and analyzing the differences.[25] In that study, joints were divided in multiple areas according to previous literature and in a reproducible way (as an example: the ankle in nine regions, the talonavicular joint in six regions, and the calcaneocuboid joint in four regions). Interestingly, the investigators were able to identify statistically significant differences in multiple areas of the above-mentioned joints. Once further studies have been published in this area, defining normal and pathologic values for each joint, it will be possible to apply DM in daily practice and to obtain immediately a much more objective assessment of joints with a quantitative analysis of its different parts. This could help identify specific overloaded areas and plan realignment procedures, which represent a cornerstone in the surgical correction of cavovarus feet.

DISCUSSION

To simplify, it could be said that cavovarus feet need to be assessed both in terms of soft tissues (in particular tendons and ligaments) and osteoarticular structure (osteology and arthrology).

The physical examination provides crucial data on tendon function and potential imbalance. As a reminder, it is common to find weakness in eversion (reduced function of the peroneus brevis tendon) and in dorsiflexion (reduced function of the tibialis anterior tendon). On the contrary, the peroneus longus and the tibialis posterior tendon keep working (increasing the cavus shape of the foot and the tendency to invert the hindfoot, respectively) with a relative overactivity as compared with their antagonist. The extensor hallux longus and extensor digitorum longus are often overcontracted to compensate the lack of activity of the tibialis anterior and provide some ability to dorsiflex the foot and reduce the steppage during the gait. Finally, the Achilles tendon, which in itself it is generally not among the initial drivers of the deformity, also becomes relatively short, with a subsequent equinus of the foot. What is more, once the hindfoot has assumed a varus configuration, the triceps surae further shortens and adapts to this new situation, therefore becoming an obstacle itself to the realignment of the heel. All these clinical data are a great help to guide the clinician in the decision about the necessity to balance tendons during surgery.

On the other side, the two main parameters which are necessary for decision-making are (1) the malalignment and (2) the joint status. With regard to malalignment, a standing tomographic imaging is needed to quantify the deformity in terms of axes and angles. This quantification is currently carried out by applying classical measurements (ie, 2D measurements) to single slices from WBCT images (both manually[12] or automatically through dedicated software[16]) or, at best, using 3D semiautomatic measurements such as the Foot and Ankle Offset first described in 2017.[26] Although the latter considers the whole deformity establishing a relationship between the center of rotation of the ankle and the Kapandji foot tripod, it does not provide sublevel information about where the deformity occurs. From this standpoint, it is crucial to consider the concept of center of rotation and angulation (CORA), which ideally applies to any type of angular deformity and is often advocated by knee surgeons to plan femur of tibia osteotomies to offload the medial of lateral compartment of the tibiofemoral joint. A quick review of the literature using the keywords "(center) AND (rotation) AND (angulation) AND (foot)" reveals that this principle has been applied mainly to hallux valgus[27,28] and supramalleolar osteotomies.[29,30] Of note, in a cadaveric study by Mortimer and colleagues, a "foot-CORA" method has been reported,[31] according to which the investigators identified the medial cuneiform as the main site of most midfoot and forefoot deformities and proposing it as target for realignment procedures. In their study, the investigators underlined the biplanar effect of medial cuneiform osteotomy demonstrating that a transverse plane correction was always (and unintentionally) associated to the sagittal correction of the foot.[31] Although the present work is focused on the imaging and not on the pathophysiology of cavovarus feet, we believe paramount to remind that these deformities represent one of the best examples of multi-CORA condition with an altered arthrology and osteology. As a matter of fact, with regard to joints: (1) the talus is internally rotated, supinated, and dorsi-flexed (or plantar-flexed in equinus feet) as compared with the tibioperoneal mortise, as the patient naturally tries to walk with a straight foot, this translates into an external rotation of the leg; (2) at the subtalar joint, the calcaneus tends to supinate itself and become more parallel to the talus, with a reduction of the kite angle; (3) at the Chopart joint, the navicular moves medially as compared with the talar head increasing the adduction and supination of the midfoot; and (4) at the midfoot the cuneiforms plantar-flex in relation to the navicular and the medial metatarsals plantarflex in relation to the cuneiforms, in particular, the first metatarsal suffers the relative overactivity of the per-oneus longus, with a subsequent pronation of the forefoot which becomes a supinated forefoot when the five metatarsal heads meet the ground and adapt to it. Regarding bony changes, we have discussed above the findings from a previous study where changes in the osteology of CMT patients have been demonstrated as compared with normal feet.[17]

Bearing these elements in mind, the investigators deem that the use of WBCT in clinical daily practice is paramount in cavovarus feet for at least two reasons: first, although bony changes might potentially be assessed on traditional CTs, it is obvious that the relationship between axes and articular surfaces of adjacent joints could be correctly assessed exclusively on images taken in weight-bearing position, which is crucial for a more accurate understanding of the deformity; second, although the cur-rent algorithms of treatment for supple deformities generally include calcaneal osteot-omies associated to dorsiflexion osteotomies of the forefoot, it is clear that they represent an attempt to restore a global mechanical balance of the foot rather than aiming to correct the CORA (or CORAs) of the deformity, which is a limitation of these surgical procedure and which could potentially explain some failures. The use of WBCT imaging could be the key to assess more accurately these deformities and hy-pothetically plan dedicated corrections to target the true CORA or CORAs case by case. This would require multiple procedures at different levels of the foot with impor-tant challenges in terms of fixation of each realigned segment and stress for soft tis-sues. Patient-specific instrumentation and 3D printing might play an important role in this setting.

SUMMARY

Cavovarus foot is a complex 3D deformity, which includes a wide range of clinical con-ditions from subtle deformities to disabling feet. The more severe such conditions are the more 2D radiographic biases hinder a correct evaluation of bones and joints. The advent of WBCT might enable to avoid double imaging (radiographs + tomography) and delays in all patients for which a detailed osteoarticular assessment is required, with the advantage to obtain 3D images in standing position and a reduction of the ra-diation exposure and time to diagnosis. Automatic measurements are being devel-oped and along with techniques to assess the joint status (such as DM) will likely allow to obtain an accurate assessment of a cavovarus foot in clinical practice to define the CORA or CORAs and to plan surgery based on a strong rationale with the aim to improve clinical outcomes.

CLINICS CARE POINTS

- Providing surgeons and patients with 3D cone beam WBCT in the context of cavovarus feet helps better understand the deformity.

- Although measurements performed 'by hand' on conventional radiographs are considered the 'gold standard', some literature challenges them demonstrating a mismatch with angles measured automatically on images from WBCT.
- The 2 main parameters for decision making in cavovarus deformity are: malalignment and joint status. Both may be accurately assessed on WBCT images, but not using the conventional radiography-MDCT sequence given the number of biases related to radiographs and the absence of load bearing during MDCT.

DISCLOSURE

F. Lintz: CURVEBEAM AI (paid consultant and stock options); President of the International Weightbearing CT Society. A. Bernasconi: CURVEBEAM AI (stock options); Board Member of the International Weightbearing CT Society; Chair of the Youth Committee of the European Foot and Ankle Society.

REFERENCES

1. Kaplan JRM, Aiyer A, Cerrato RA, et al. Operative Treatment of the Cavovarus Foot. Foot Ankle Int 2018;39(11):1370–82.
2. Aminian A, Sangeorzan BJ. The anatomy of cavus foot deformity. Foot Ankle Clin 2008;13(2):191–8, v.
3. Maynou C, Szymanski C, Thiounn A. The adult cavus foot. EFORT Open Rev 2017;2(5):221–9.
4. Manoli A, Graham B. The subtle cavus foot, "the underpronator". Foot Ankle Int 2005;26(3):256–63.
5. Baverel L, Brilhault J, Odri G, et al. Influence of lower limb rotation on hindfoot alignment using a conventional two-dimensional radiographic technique. Foot Ankle Surg 2017;23(1):44–9.
6. Willauer P, Sangeorzan BJ, Whittaker EC, et al. The sensitivity of standard radiographic foot measures to misalignment. Foot Ankle Int 2014;35(12):1334–40.
7. Bernasconi A, de Cesar Netto C, Barg A, et al. AAFD: Conventional Radiographs are not Enough! i Need the Third Dimension. Tech Foot Ankle Surg 2019;18(3).
8. Saltzman CL, El-Khoury GY. The Hindfoot Alignment View. Foot Ankle Int 1995; 16(9):572–6.
9. Reilingh ML, Beimers L, Tuijthof GJM, et al. Measuring hindfoot alignment radiographically: the long axial view is more reliable than the hindfoot alignment view. Skeletal Radiol 2010;39(11):1103–8.
10. Lintz F, Netto C de C, Barg A, et al. Weight-bearing cone beam CT scans in the foot and ankle. EFORT Open Rev 2018;3(5):278–86.
11. Godoy-Santos A,A, Bernasconi A, Bordalo-Rodrigues M, et al. Weight-bearing cone-beam computed tomography in the foot and ankle specialty: where we are and where we are going - an update. Radiol Bras 2021;54(3):177–84.
12. Bernasconi A, Cooper L, Lyle S, et al. Intraobserver and interobserver reliability of cone beam weightbearing semi-automatic three-dimensional measurements in symptomatic pes cavovarus. Foot Ankle Surg 2019. https://doi.org/10.1016/j.fas.2019.07.005.
13. Bernasconi A, Cooper L, Lyle S, et al. Pes cavovarus in Charcot-Marie-Tooth compared to the idiopathic cavovarus foot: A preliminary weightbearing CT analysis. Foot Ankle Surg 2020. https://doi.org/10.1016/j.fas.2020.04.004.

14. An T, Haupt E, Michalski M, et al. Cavovarus With a Twist: Midfoot Coronal and Axial Plane Rotational Deformity in Charcot-Marie-Tooth Disease. Foot Ankle Int 2022;43(5):676–82.

15. Richter M, Duerr F, Schilke R, et al. Semi-automatic software-based 3D-angular measurement for Weight-Bearing CT (WBCT) in the foot provides different angles than measurement by hand. Foot Ankle Surg 2022;28(7):919–27.

16. Sangoi D, Ranjit S, Bernasconi A, et al. 2D Manual vs 3D Automated Assessment of Alignment in Normal and Charcot-Marie-Tooth Cavovarus Feet Using Weight-bearing CT. Foot Ankle Int 2022;43(7):973–82.

17. Michalski MP, An TW, Haupt ET, et al. Abnormal Bone Morphology in Charcot-Marie-Tooth Disease. Foot Ankle Int 2022;43(4):576–81.

18. Vier D, Louis T, Fuchs D, et al. Radiographic assessment of the subtalar joint: An evaluation of the Kellgren-Lawrence scale and proposal of a novel scale. Clin Imaging 2020;60(1):62–6.

19. Mayich DJ, Pinsker E, Mayich MS, et al. An analysis of the use of the Kellgren and Lawrence grading system to evaluate peritalar arthritis following total ankle arthroplasty. Foot Ankle Int 2013;34(11):1508–15.

20. Siegler S, Konow T, Belvedere C, et al. Analysis of surface-to-surface distance mapping during three-dimensional motion at the ankle and subtalar joints. J Biomech 2018;76:204–11.

21. Corazza F, Stagni R, Castelli VP, et al. Articular contact at the tibiotalar joint in passive flexion. J Biomech 2005;38(6):1205–12.

22. Bernasconi A, de Cesar Netto C, Siegler S, et al. Weightbearing CT assessment of foot and ankle joints in Pes Planovalgus using distance mapping. Foot Ankle Surg 2022;28(6):775–84.

23. Dibbern KN, Li S, Vivtcharenko V, et al. Three-Dimensional Distance and Coverage Maps in the Assessment of Peritalar Subluxation in Progressive Collapsing Foot Deformity. Foot Ankle Int 2021;42(6):757–67.

24. Behrens A, Dibbern K, Lalevée M, et al. Coverage maps demonstrate 3D Chopart joint subluxation in weightbearing CT of progressive collapsing foot deformity. Sci Rep 2022;12(1). https://doi.org/10.1038/S41598-022-23638-3.

25. Lintz F, Jepsen M, de Cesar Netto C, et al. Distance mapping of the foot and ankle joints using weightbearing CT: The cavovarus configuration. Foot Ankle Surg 2020. https://doi.org/10.1016/j.fas.2020.05.007.

26. Lintz F, Welck M, Bernasconi A, et al. 3D Biometrics for Hindfoot Alignment Using Weightbearing CT. Foot Ankle Int 2017;38(6). https://doi.org/10.1177/107110071 7690806.

27. Wagner E, Ortiz C, Wagner P. Using the Center of Rotation of Angulation Concept in Hallux Valgus Correction: Why Do We Choose the Proximal Oblique Sliding Closing Wedge Osteotomy? Foot Ankle Clin 2018;23(2):247–56.

28. Mashima N, Yamamoto H, Tsuboi I, et al. Correction of hallux valgus deformity using the center of rotation of angulation method. J Orthop Sci 2009;14(4):377–84.

29. Mendicino RW, Catanzariti AR, Reeves CL. Percutaneous supramalleolar osteotomy for distal tibial (near articular) ankle deformities. J Am Podiatr Med Assoc 2005;95(1):72–84.

30. Al-Nammari SS, Myerson MS. The Use of Tibial Osteotomy (Ankle Plafondplasty) for Joint Preservation of Ankle Deformity and Early Arthritis. Foot Ankle Clin 2016; 21(1):15–26.

31. Mortimer JA, Bouchard M, Acosta A, et al. The Biplanar Effect of the Medial Cuneiform Osteotomy. Foot Ankle Spec 2020;13(3):250–7.

Is Subtle Cavovarus a Problem for Athletes?

Ashraf T. Hantouly, MD, MSc[a], Ahmed Khalil Attia, MD, PGDipClinEd[b],
Khalid Hasan, MD, MPH[c], Pieter D'Hooghe, MD, PhD[d],*

KEYWORDS

- Athletes • Ankle sprains • Foot biomechanics • Metatarsal fracture
- Subtle cavovarus • Peroneal tendon injury

KEY POINTS

- Subtle cavovarus foot (SCF), the mild form of cavus foot, is a common pathology that is usually underreported.
- A careful clinical examination is required to diagnose SCF and its associated conditions.
- SCF has a significant impact on the athletic population due to the associated conditions such as chronic ankle pain, ankle instability, metatarsals stress fractures, and peroneal tendons pathology.
- Addressing the anatomical abnormality of the cavus foot is substantial for proper treatment of the associated conditions.

INTRODUCTION

Cavovarus or high-arched foot is a common foot deformity that occurs due to the disruption of the foot-driven equilibrium between the first metatarsal, fifth metatarsal, and the heel. This imbalance leads to an increase in the foot's normal plantar concavity. Cavovarus deformity ranges from a mild and flexible malalignment to a fixed, complex, and severe deformation.

Subtle cavovarus foot (SCF), the mild form of the cavus foot, was first described by Manoli and his colleagues.[1] Since then, it has been increasingly accepted to be identified as an idiopathic non-neurogenic cause of cavus foot. This deformity is characterized by mild heel varus, forefoot pronation, and plantarflexion of the first ray.

SCF can negatively impact patients especially the athletic population as this set of patients are of high demand and prone to repetitive injuries. These patients may experience chronic pain, instability, recurrent injuries, and balance issues. However,

[a] Department of Orthopedic Surgery, Hamad Medical Corporation, Doha 3050, Qatar;
[b] Department of Orthopaedic Surgery, University of Pittsburgh, Pittsburgh, PA, USA; [c] Virginia Commonwealth University, 1200 East Broad Street, 9th Floor, Richmond, VA 23298, USA;
[d] Aspetar Orthopaedic and Sports Medicine Hospital, Doha, Qatar
* Corresponding author. Sportscity Street 1, PO Box 29222, Aspire Zone, Aspetar Hospital, Doha, Qatar.
E-mail address: Pieter.orthopedie@gmail.com

Foot Ankle Clin N Am 28 (2023) 729–741
https://doi.org/10.1016/j.fcl.2023.05.010
1083-7515/23/© 2023 Elsevier Inc. All rights reserved.

despite the high prevalence of SCF, there is scarce evidence on its impact on the athletic population and its associated injuries.

To bridge this gap, the authors aimed to synthesize the current evidence and provide a comprehensive review on SCFs effects on athletes. Furthermore, this article explains SCF biomechanics and highlights its commonly associated injuries and their management.

BIOMECHANICS: RISK OF INJURY

Pes cavus or cavus foot is a spectrum of deformity commonly faced by foot and ankle surgeons. The use of the term pes cavus dates back to 1885 by Shaffer MD. It has been reported that up to 15% of the population has cavovarus foot.[2] Anatomically, the deformity can be described as a combination of the following components.[3,4]

- High longitudinal plantar arch
- Varus heel alignment
- High calcaneal pitch
- High midfoot pitch
- Equinus, pronation, and adduction of the forefoot
- Plantarflexion of the first ray.

The deformity can be either forefoot or hindfoot driven.[3,5,6] Neurologic diseases leading to muscle imbalance are common in forefoot-related cavus foot deformity. The peroneus longus and tibialis posterior tendon overpower the peroneus brevis and tibialis anterior tendon leading to the typical cavovarus foot. The main underlying reason for the hindfoot-driven cavus can be attributed to a sequela of a traumatic injury.[4] Nevertheless, a variety of underlying factors has been described in the literature.[1,7] It is imperative to comprehend certain biomechanics of the gait cycle to appreciate the risk of injury in athletes with an SCF. The gait is broadly divided into stance and swing phases.[8] The locking and unlocking mechanism of Chopart joint plays an integral part of the gait cycle.[3] The heel is everted at the end of the stance phase and inverted at the heel strike and midstance stages. During the unlocked phase, the calcaneocuboid and talonavicular joints are parallel, which allows for motion at the Chopart joint leading to a flexible hindfoot and the ability to absorb shock. During the locked phase, these joints are not parallel and therefore stabilize the midfoot. This rigidity helps in push-off and forward propulsion.[3,9–11]

In cavovarus foot, altered gait mechanisms have been reported in multiple studies. The heel does not evert normally at the end of the stance phase. Moreover, the plantar-flexed first ray hits the ground before the heel can fully evert. This leads to decreased absorption of shock at heel strike, uneven loading of bony structures with overloading of the lateral foot and ankle and therefore weakening of the lateral soft tissue structures over time.[12–15] The muscle imbalance also plays a significant role in the altered biomechanics as the peroneus longus overpowering plantar flexes the first ray prematurely locking the Chopart joint earlier in the gait cycle.[16] As the lateral structures attenuate, it causes the pressure to increase on the medial structures as well as contractures of the medial structures.[17,18]

Cavovarus deformity can range from flexible to rigid. As the deformity progresses, it can enter a vicious cycle of abnormal biomechanics. As the first ray becomes more rigid and stays plantar-flexed, continually forcing the heel into varus. Over time, once the hindfoot becomes rigid, gastrocnemius contracts and it makes the Achilles tendon a secondary invertor hence accentuating the problem.[19,20] These altered biomechanics in the SCF put the athletes at a higher risk of injury and associated pathologies.[21,22]

SPORTS INJURIES RELATED TO CAVOVARUS

SCF causes medial displacement of the mechanical axis of the lower limb and uneven distribution of the load pressure during the gait cycle, which disrupts the biomechanics of the leg, ankle, and foot. This, in turn, creates excessive medial compressive forces and lateral tensile forces[18,23] that disrupt the integrity of the surrounding anatomical structures leading to wide arrays of conditions affecting the entire lower limb.[23] Athletes with SCF are prone to a higher incidence of lateral ankle pain, metatarsalgia, stress fractures, ankle sprains, chronic lateral ankle instability (CLAI), peroneal tendon injuries, foot calluses, plantar fasciitis, Achilles tendonitis, lateral foot ulcers, or even ankle and midfoot arthritis.[24] **Box 1** lists the various conditions associated with SCF.[24,25]

PERONEAL TENDONS PATHOLOGIES

Peroneal tendons are major dynamic stabilizers and the primary evertors of the ankle. Owing to their anatomic and histologic structure, they have limited ability to compensate for length changes. The peroneal longus is a bipennate muscle with short tendon excursion, and therefore, partial or even full-thickness tears might result from small changes in its resting length. Moreover, even small tears can significantly alter the tendons' biomechanics and function as ankle stabilizers.[26] Therefore, a subtle change in the normal anatomy, such as SCF, might trigger various spectrum of peroneal tendons pathologies.

Pathologic abnormalities of these tendons account for a significant proportion of ankle and lateral hindfoot dysfunction. These pathologies can be categorized into three main types: tendinitis, subluxation/dislocation, and splits/tears (**Fig. 1**).[27] Peroneal tendon pathologies have been linked to anatomic abnormalities, ankle instability,

---

Box 1
Subtle cavovarus foot-associated conditions[24,25]

Foot and ankle conditions
    Chronic ankle pain
    Ankle instability
    Subtalar instability
    Peroneus brevis and longus split
    Peroneal tendons subluxation/dislocation
    Os peroneum syndrome
    Enlarged peroneal tubercle
    Fifth metatarsal base fracture
    Fourth metatarsal base fracture
    Callus under the first and fifth metatarsal heads
    Callus under the fifth metatarsal base
    Sesamoiditis, sesamoid chondromalacia, and avascular necrosis
    Plantar fasciitis
    Ankle arthritis
    Midfoot arthritis

Other associated conditions
    Knee arthritis
    Iliotibial band syndrome
    Tibia and fibula stress fractures
    Leg exertional compartment syndrome

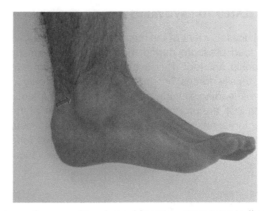

Fig. 1. Clinical picture of peroneal tendon subluxation. Foot is typically examined in active dorsiflexion and eversion against resistance (apprehension test).

and repetitive inversion injuries. It has been reported that such pathologies are found in up to 77% of patients with ankle instability and 4% of all ankle injuries.[28,29] Moreover, it has been shown that peroneal tendon tears are highly linked to cavovarus foot as Brandes and colleagues reported that cavovarus was found in 82% of their operatively treated peroneal tears.[26] Despite these numbers, only 60% of peroneal pathologies are accurately detected.[30]

Symptoms of peroneal injuries range from lateral ankle/foot pain, swelling, and weakness to ankle instability and reparative ankle sprains that hinder the athlete's ability to participate in physical activities. Consequently, due to the high mechanical loads exerted on the peroneal tendons, they are prone to hypertrophic tendinopathy, stenosis, subluxation, dislocation, and tearing.[23,27,31]

Management of peroneal tendon pathologies requires careful attention, a systematic examination and accurate diagnosis. Moreover, identifying the underlying etiology, especially the SCF, is crucial for proper management. Treating these pathologies depends on the stage and chronicity of the disease. The spectrum ranges from conservative management (rest, activity modification, nonsteroidal anti-inflammatory medications) to surgical management that is tailored to the underlying pathology. This includes synovectomy, tendon repair/reconstruction/rerouting, retromalleolar groove deepening, distal fibula bone-block procedures, and hindfoot varus correction with calcaneal and first metatarsal osteotomies.[23,27,31]

Conservative management of peroneal subluxation has been proven to have inferior outcomes, especially in the athletic population. Therefore, surgical intervention has been adopted as the standard of care in acute subluxation in this group of patients.[32] A meta-analysis, which included 12 studies investigating peroneal tendons subluxation/dislocation, showed that surgical management of such injuries results in high satisfaction rate and low re-dislocation rate (<1.5%). They also found that superior peroneal retinaculum repair associated with retromalleolar groove deepening had satisfactory outcomes and high return to play (RTP) rate.[33]

ANKLE SPRAINS AND CHRONIC LATERAL ANKLE INSTABILITY

Ankle sprains are the most common ankle injury with inversion injuries being the most common. Most of these sprains respond well to a period of brief immobilization and functional rehabilitation. Nonetheless, about 20% of these sprains progress to mechanical or functional instability.[34] The relationship between cavovarus foot align-ment and ankle sprains and instability has been well-documented for decades.[35] Strauss and colleagues reported on associated extra-articular conditions in 160 an-kles with CLAI.[36] They found the prevalence of hindfoot varus alignment to be 8% of ankles with CLAI and 28% of revision lateral ankle ligament repairs. They reported that failure to correct hindfoot varus was the most common cause of failure of surgical intervention.[36] Larsen and Angermann compared 95 patients undergoing surgery for lateral ankle instability with a control group. They found that the surgical group had an increased arch height on weight-bearing lateral films.[37] A study by Van Bergeyk and colleagues used simulated weight-bearing CT scans to show that patients with CLAI have increased heel calcaneal varus in comparison to controls.[38]

Nonoperative management should focus on proprioception and peroneal strengthening. Although subtle cavovarus does not have a neurologic cause, sub-clinical muscle imbalance may be present in these patients. Recovery from an ankle sprain and prevention of recurrence depends on accurate proprioceptive and neuro-muscular control.[39] In addition, orthotics can be vital for satisfactory outcomes and are well-tolerated. In terms of surgical management for CLAI with subtle cavovarus in athletes, Broström anatomic repair with suture tape augmentation is recommen-ded. Postoperatively, orthotics to correct the foot alignment should be used throughout the recovery and athletic activities. In revision cases, in addition to the above, a calcaneal osteotomy can be added to correct the hindfoot alignment and reduce the risk of recurrent sprains. Unfortunately, studies on outcomes of lat-eralizing calcaneal osteotomies in athletes with ankle sprains and concomitant hind-foot varus are limited in the literature with most studies reporting on the general population. Vienne and colleagues reported on nine ankles in eight patients with cavovarus who failed lateral ankle stabilization surgery.[40] In their study, all patients underwent lateral displacement calcaneal osteotomy and peroneus longus to pero-neus brevis tendon transfer. They reported clinical and radiological improvement af-ter deformity correction.[40] Fortin and colleagues reported on the management of CLAI with idiopathic cavovarus deformity.[41] In their study, few patients underwent a calcaneal osteotomy. However, they concluded that the correction of cavovarus deformity may aid in balancing the forces across the ankle and improving the effec-tiveness of a lateral ligament repair.[41] A study by Shim and colleagues reported on 15 cases of CLAI and subtle varus with a peek-a-poo heel sign.[42] Seven patients (46.7%) had a calcaneal lateral closing wedge osteotomy, and the first metatarsal dorsiflexion osteotomy was performed in 11 patients (73.3%). Three patients (20%) underwent both osteotomies. The choice for surgery was guided by the re-sults of the Coleman block test. They reported significant improvement in both func-tional and radiographic parameters with no recurrence of CLAI at a mean follow-up of 58 months.[42]

In summary, the decision for calcaneal and/or first metatarsal osteotomy should be individualized, and every attempt to avoid changing the foot mechanics in high-level athletes should be made unless absolutely indicated. Generally, osteotomies should be avoided in primary cases with subtle deformity and reserved for revisions and large deformities. If lateralizing calcaneal osteotomy is indicated, a minimally invasive sur-gery (MIS) approach using burrs and percutaneous fixation can be extremely valuable to avoid the rather large lateral incision of the open procedure that is typically in close proximity to that of the Broström procedure. The MIS osteotomy becomes even more valuable if peroneal tendons work is to be done as well. Finally, if a calcaneal osteot-omy is planned, soft tissue imbrication should be done after the osteotomy is fixed to ensure maximal tension of the lateral soft tissues.

JONES FRACTURE

Jones fractures are fifth metatarsal base fractures at the meta-diaphyseal junction. They are named after Sir Robert Jones who sustained the fracture himself while dancing in 1902.[43] Many if not most of these fractures are stress fractures with prodromal symptoms for extended periods.[44,45] The mechanism of injury in acute fractures is believed to be a considerable adduction force applied to a plantar-flexed ankle with most of the body weight on the metatarsal heads.[46] These forces are possibly exacerbated by unaddressed underlying altered foot mechanics such as cavovarus, metatarsus adductus, or a prominent fifth metatarsal head.[47] The rationale is that cavus feet are relatively rigid and unable to absorb the high repetitive forces experienced by the foot, placing increased lateral loads on the lateral structures of the foot including the fifth metatarsal base.[48–50] The meta-diaphyseal junction represents a transition between the stiff proximal fifth metatarsal with insertions of the peroneus brevis and plantar aponeurosis and the highly mobile fifth ray.

The association between cavovarus feet and Jones fractures has been well reported. In a study by Lee and colleagues, the investigators reported an increased association between cavus feet and jones fractures.[51] In another study, the National Football League (NFL) combine database was reviewed and 74 fractures were identified in 68 players.[52] Coronal plane alignment, as measured by talar first metatarsal angle, talar-second metatarsal angle, and talar-fifth MT angle, showed significant differences between the fracture and control groups, with a higher incidence of Jones fractures in athletes who had cavovarus feet.[52] Raikin and colleagues reported on 21 Jones fractures in 20 athletes treated with intramedullary screw fixation. They found 18 out of 21 feet to be in varus. They recommended orthotics to correct the malignant as a part of their postoperative regimen.[45]

Management of primary Jones fractures in athletes with cavus feet follows the same principles as in those with neutral and valgus alignment. Surgical management of all jones fractures in athletes is strongly recommended.[47] In a recent meta-analysis of 22 studies by Attia and colleagues, surgical management of Jones fractures using intramedullary screw fixation led to a 98.8% RTP rate in comparison to 71.6% in those treated conservatively.[47] They also reported a higher union rate and faster union with surgical management.[47] Postoperatively, the correction of the foot alignment using custom-made stiff orthotics with first metatarsal head recess and lateral heel post is recommended (**Fig. 2**).

Despite the excellent RTP rates, returning to the previous level of participation can be lengthy. Spang and colleagues in their study of the NFL Scouting Combine reported that players with Jones fractures had a worse performance for the following two seasons in comparison with that of controls.[53] They also found that the number of cortices that were united on CT was correlated with performance. The investigators used snap counts, defined as the total number of plays in which a player participated out of the total number of plays in which the player was eligible to participate throughout a season. Almost all player positions showed statistically significant lower scores in comparison with controls, with running backs having the worst participation among all positions.[53]

Despite the excellent outcomes of intramedullary (IM) screw fixation for Jones fractures, refractures remain common and can affect up to 10% after complete fracture union.[47] This is especially true if the malalignment is not corrected. In revision cases for refractures, there is limited evidence on whether a calcaneal osteotomy is indicated in subtle cavus feet in athletes. Granata and colleagues reported on 4 refractures out of 55 Jones fractures. One of these four refractures required a Dwyer calcaneal osteotomy for varus malalignment in addition to revision IM screw fixation.[54]

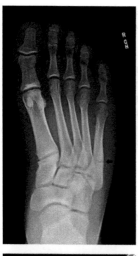
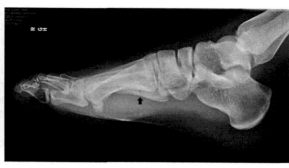
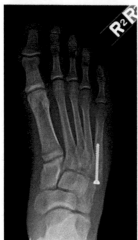
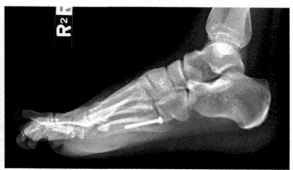

Fig. 2. Preoperative (top) and 4 weeks postoperative (bottom) plain films of a 20-year-old college football player with varus hindfoot and metatarsus adductus who sustained an acute Jones fracture (*arrow*). He underwent intramedullary screw fixation with a chamfered 4.5 mm solid cancellous screw and bone marrow aspirate concentrate (BMAC) injection.

In summary, a thorough clinical examination and an early recognition of prodromal symptoms in cavovarus foot remain crucial. A high index of suspicion and a low threshold for MR imaging should be exercised in athletes with cavus feet who present with lateral foot pain. In addition to IM screw fixation, rigid custom-made orthotics is essential. Athletes should not be allowed to RTP without radiographic evidence of complete union on CT scan. A calcaneal osteotomy should be reserved for revision cases and decided on a case-to-case basis.

ACHILLES TENDON

Achilles tendon pathologies are not uncommon in athletes with subtle cavovarus feet. Gastrocnemius or Achilles tendon tightness is a usual clinical finding.[55] As the cavovarus deformity becomes more rigid, it forces the heel to permanently stay in a varus position. This, along with contracted medial structures, causes the gastrocnemius muscle and Achilles tendon to contract over period resulting in Achilles tendon becoming a strong invertor.[19,20]

Insertional Achilles tendinitis also often develops over time. This occurs as the posterior superior calcaneal tuberosity becomes more prominent due to the heel being in varus and Achilles or gastrocnemius tightness.[20] One of the mainstays of nonoperative treatment is gastrocnemius stretching program to address the tightness.[39] Likewise, Achilles tendon lengthening is an important component of the cavovarus deformity reconstruction. This can be performed effectively in a percutaneous or minimally invasive manner.

MINIMALLY INVASIVE SURGERY VERSUS OPEN

MIS versus open surgery in athletes with SCF can be broadly divided into treatment of injuries versus reconstruction of deformity. Following are some of the most common injuries/problems that may require surgical treatment.[24]

- Fifth metatarsal fractures
- Lateral ankle instability
- Osteochondral lesions (OCL) of ankle
- Plantar fasciitis
- Achilles tendonitis and rupture
- Peroneal tendinitis and tear

Cavovarus foot deformity is one of the significant risk factors for sustaining a fifth metatarsal base fracture.[55] The standard of treatment for the fifth metatarsal base fractures in athletes is a single intramedullary screw which is done with a small incision.[48,56] Excellent union rate has been demonstrated in literature with this technique even in patients with cavovarus foot deformity.[45] Open reduction and internal fixation have typically been reserved for recurrent fractures and nonunion.

CLAI is frequently seen in athletes with SCF.[37] The modified Brostrom procedure has been noted to be an effective method in treating lateral ankle instability with excellent results.[57,58] The repair can be performed arthroscopically or in an open fashion. Both methods for lateral ankle ligamentous reconstruction have been studied extensively. Arthroscopic surgery has shown superior results compared with open repair in a recent systematic review and meta-analysis.[34]

Athletes with subtle cavovarus feet are more prone to ankle sprains; they are also at a higher risk of developing OCL of the talus.[59] Surgical treatment of osteochondral lesions of talus (OLT) can be performed arthroscopically versus open depending on the lesion stage, size, location, and surgeons' experience.[60–62] It has been suggested that the OLT lesions should be treated in similar fashion irrespective of the alignment of the ankle and foot.[63]

Plantar fasciitis in athletes with SCF results as a sequela of foot rigidity and inability to disperse forces.[64] It usually occurs in conjunction with tight gastrocnemius–soleus complex. Although the foremost treatment for plantar fasciitis is mostly nonoperative, plantar fascia release can be performed for recalcitrant cases. Studies have shown equivalent results with open versus percutaneous or endoscopic plantar fascial release.[65] Similarly, Achilles tendon lengthening and gastrocnemius release can be performed in a percutaneous or endoscopically with good results.

SCF is an acknowledged reason for Achilles tendonitis and rupture injuries.[66] Tightness and chronic irritation of the Achilles tendon as a result of the SCF deformity have been well-described in the literature.[20] Minimally invasive treatment for Achilles tendon rupture has demonstrated a lower risk of infection and wound complications but on the expense of a higher risk of iatrogenic nerve damage.[67,68]

Open visualization of tendons and surgical treatment has been the mainstay for peroneal tendon pathologies once the conservative measures have failed. Several small-sized studies where endoscopic-assisted synovectomy, tenodesis, and retromalleolar groove deepening have been performed successfully with satisfactory results.[69,70]

Surgical correction of cavovarus foot deformity depends on the degree of muscle imbalance and structural deformities. The primary aim of surgical fixation is to obtain a stable plantigrade foot. There are several components to performing a cavovarus foot deformity correction.[20]

- Soft tissue procedures
- Osteotomies
- Arthrodesis
- Tendon transfers
- Correction of structural deformities

Soft tissue procedures including Achilles tendon lengthening, plantar fascia release, deltoid ligament release, and lateral ligament reconstruction can be performed in an open fashion or MIS. As mentioned earlier, osteotomies should be avoided in primary cases with subtle deformity and reserved for more complex deformities. However, if lateralizing calcaneal osteotomy is indicated, the MIS approach has been proven to be highly valuable. Moreover, first-ray dorsiflexion and midtarsal closing wedge osteotomies have been successfully performed with the MIS technique, but there have been concerns that biomechanical fundamentals of deformity correction are undermined with MIS for a smaller scar and marketing reasons.[71] Arthroscopy-assisted arthrodesis in the foot and ankle is well-defined and has resulted in excellent results.[72]

Cavovarus foot deformity may require peroneus longus tendon transfer to peroneus brevis, posterior tibial tendon transfer to dorsum of foot, anterior tibial tendon transfer to the middle of the foot, and extensor hallucis longus transfer to first metatarsal depending on the degree of muscle imbalance. Percutaneous and minimally invasive techniques have been well described for tendon transfers in foot and ankle and can be applied successfully in reconstruction of cavovarus foot.[73]

SUMMARY

- SCF deformity is a common foot deformity that is defined as an idiopathic non-neurogenic mild form of cavus foot.
- SCF anatomical deformity is a combination of high longitudinal plantar arch, varus heel alignment, high calcaneal pitch, high midfoot pitch, equinus, pronation, and adduction of the forefoot and plantarflexion of the first ray.
- SCF negatively impacts athletes and increases their risk of developing lateral ankle pain, recurrent ankle sprains, CLAI, peroneal tendon injuries, foot calluses, plantar fasciitis, metatarsalgia, stress fractures, Achilles tendonitis, lateral foot ulcers, or even ankle and midfoot arthritis.
- Peroneal tendon pathologies can be categorized into three main types: (1) tendinitis, (2) subluxation/dislocation, and (3) splits/tears.
- Nonoperative management of ankle sprains associated with SCF should focus on proprioception exercises, neuromuscular control, and peroneal strengthening, in addition to the use of orthotics.

- Brostrom anatomic repair with suture augmentation is recommended for chronic ankle instability in the athletic population, and calcaneal osteotomies are preserved for revision cases.
- A high index of suspicion and a low threshold for MRI should be exercised in athletes with cavus feet who present with lateral foot pain to rule out Jones fracture.
- Intramedullary screw is the recommended management of Jones fracture in the athletes. It results in higher union rates, shorter time to union, and greater than 98% RTP. However, athletes tend to have a worse performance for the following two seasons.
- The mainstays of the conservative treatment of Achilles tendon tightness is gastrocnemius stretching programs. However, Achilles tendon lengthening is an important component of the cavovarus deformity reconstruction.
- The MIS approach is a highly valuable technique to address SCF deformity and its associated conditions.

DECLARATIONS

- *Conflicts of interest* Authors declare that they have no conflict of interest.
- *Consent to participate* Not applicable.
- *Consent for publication* Not applicable.
- *Ethical approval* This article does not contain any studies with human participants performed by any of the authors.
- *Funding* There is no funding source.
- *Code availability* Not applicable
- *Availability of data and material* Not applicable

REFERENCES

1. Deben SE, Pomeroy GC. Subtle Cavus Foot. J Am Acad Orthop Surg 2014;22(8): 512–20.
2. Walker M, Fan HJ. Relationship Between Foot Pressure Pattern and Foot Type. Foot Ankle Int 1998;19(6):379–83.
3. Apostle KL, Sangeorzan BJ. Anatomy of the Varus Foot and Ankle. Foot Ankle Clin 2012;17(1):1–11.
4. Krähenbühl N, Weinberg MW. Anatomy and Biomechanics of Cavovarus Deformity. Foot Ankle Clin 2019;24(2):173–81.
5. Nogueira MP, Farcetta F, Zuccon A. Cavus Foot. Foot Ankle Clin 2015;20(4): 645–56.
6. Younger ASE, Hansen ST. Adult Cavovarus Foot. J Am Acad Orthop Surg 2005; 13(5):302–15.
7. Maskill MP, Maskill JD, Pomeroy GC. Surgical Management and Treatment Algorithm for the Subtle Cavovarus Foot. Foot Ankle Int 2010;31(12):1057–63.
8. Murray MP, Drought AB, Kory RC. Walking Patterns of Normal Men. J Bone Joint Surg Am 1994;46:335–60.
9. Sammarco VJ. The Talonavicular and Calcaneocuboid Joints: Anatomy, biomechanics, and clinical management of the transverse tarsal joint. Foot Ankle Clin 2004;9(1):127–45.
10. Manter JT. Movements of the Subtalar and Transverse Tarsal Joints. Anat Rec 1941;80(4):397–410.
11. Elftman H. The transverse tarsal joint and its control. Clin Orthop 1960;16:41–6.

12. Ledoux WR, Shofer JB, Ahroni JH, et al. Biomechanical Differences Among Pes Cavus, Neutrally Aligned, and Pes Planus Feet in Subjects with Diabetes. Foot Ankle Int 2003;24(11):845–50.

13. Cotton FJ. Foot Statics and Surgery. N Engl J Med 1936;214(8):353–62.

14. Morton DJ. The human foot: its evolution, physiology and functional disorders. Columbia University Press; 1935.

15. Mosca VS. The Cavus Foot. J Pediatr Orthop 2001;21(4):423–4.

16. Louwerens JWK, Linge B van, de Klerk LWL, et al. Peroneus Longus and Tibialis Anterior Muscle Activity in the Stance Phase: A quantified electromyographic study of 10 controls and 25 patients with chronic ankle instability. Acta Orthop Scand 1995;66(6):517–23.

17. Klammer G, Benninger E, Espinosa N. The Varus Ankle and Instability. Foot Ankle Clin 2012;17(1):57–82.

18. Krause F, Windolf M, Schwieger K, et al. Ankle Joint Pressure in Pes Cavovarus. J Bone Joint Surg Br 2007;89-B(12):1660–5.

19. Ortiz C, Wagner E, Keller A. Cavovarus Foot Reconstruction. Foot Ankle Clin 2009;14(3):471–87.

20. Kim BS. Reconstruction of Cavus Foot: A Review. Open Orthop J 2017;11(1): 651–9.

21. Williams DS III, McClay IS, Hamill J. Arch Structure and Injury Patterns in Runners. Clin BioMech 2001;16(4):341–7.

22. Cowan DN, Jones BH, Robinson JR. Foot Morphologic Characteristics and Risk of Exercise-Related Injury. Arch Fam Med 1993;2(7):773–7.

23. Abbasian A, Pomeroy G. The idiopathic Cavus Foot-not so Subtle after All. Foot Ankle Clin 2013;18(4):629–42.

24. Qin B, Wu S, Zhang H. Evaluation and Management of Cavus Foot in Adults: A Narrative Review. J Clin Med 2022;11(13):3679.

25. Manoli A 2nd, Graham B. The Subtle Cavus Foot, "the underpronator". Foot Ankle Int 2005;26(3):256–63.

26. Brandes CB, Smith RW. Characterization of Patients with Primary Peroneus Longus Tendinopathy: A review of twenty-two cases. Foot Ankle Int 2000;21(6): 462–8.

27. Davda K, Malhotra K, O'Donnell P, et al. Peroneal Tendon Disorders. EFORT Open Rev 2017;2(6):281–92.

28. DiGiovanni BF, Fraga CJ, Cohen BE, et al. Associated Injuries Found in Chronic Lateral Ankle Instability. Foot Ankle Int 2000;21:809–15.

29. Mulcahey MK, Bernhardson AS, Murphy CP, et al. The Epidemiology of Ankle Injuries Identified at the National Football League Combine, 2009–2015. Orthop J Sports Med 2018;6. 2325967118786227.

30. Dombek MF, Lamm BM, Saltrick K, et al. Peroneal Tendon Tears: A retrospective review. J Foot Ankle Surg 2003;42:250–8.

31. Van Dijk PAD, Kerkhoffs GMMJ, Chiodo C, et al. Chronic Disorders of the Peroneal Tendons: Current concepts review of the literature. J Am Acad Orthop Surg 2019;27(16):590–8.

32. Roth JA, Taylor WC, Whalen J. Peroneal Tendon Subluxation: The other lateral ankle injury. Br J Sports Med 2010;44(14):1047–53.

33. Van Dijk PA, Gianakos AL, Kerkhoffs GM, et al. Return to Sports and Clinical Outcomes in Patients Treated for Peroneal Tendon Dislocation: A systematic review. Knee Surg Sports Traumatol Arthrosc 2016;24(4):1155–64.

34. Attia AK, Taha T, Mahmoud K, et al. Outcomes of Open Versus Arthroscopic Broström Surgery for Chronic Lateral Ankle Instability: A Systematic Review and Meta-analysis of Comparative Studies. Orthop J Sports Med 2021;9(7). 23259671211015207.

35. Myerson M. Current Therapy in foot and ankle surgery. St Louis (MO): Mosby Yearbook; 1993. p. 203–9.

36. Strauss JE, Forsberg JA, Lippert FG. Chronic Lateral Ankle Instability and Associated Conditions: A rationale for treatment. Foot Ankle Int 2007;28:1041–4.

37. Larsen E, Angermann P. Association of Ankle Instability and Foot Deformity. Acta Orthop Scand 1990;61:136–9.

38. Van Bergeyk AB, Younger A, Carson B. CT Analysis of Hindfoot Alignment in Chronic Lateral Ankle Instability. Foot Ankle Int 2001;23:37–42.

39. Bosman HA, Robinson AH. Treatment of Ankle Instability with an Associated Cavus Deformity. Foot Ankle Clin 2013;18(4):643–57.

40. Vienne P, Schöniger R, Helmy N, et al. Hindfoot Instability in Cavovarus Deformity: Static and dynamic balancing. Foot Ankle Int 2007;28:96–102.

41. Fortin PT, Guettler J, Manoli A 2nd. Idiopathic Cavovarus and Lateral Ankle Instability: Recognition and treatment implications relating to ankle arthritis. Foot Ankle Int 2002;23:1031–7.

42. Shim DW, Suh JW, Park KH, et al. Diagnosis and Operation Results for Chronic Lateral Ankle Instability with Subtle Cavovarus Deformity and a Peek-A-Boo Heel Sign. Yonsei Med J 2020;61(7):635–9.

43. Jones R. I: Fracture of the Base of the Fifth Metatarsal Bone by Indirect Violence. Ann Surg 1902;35:697–702.

44. Ekstrand J, Van Dijk CN. Fifth Metatarsal Fractures Among Male Professional Footballers: A potential career-ending disease. Br J Sports Med 2013;47:754–8.

45. Raikin SM, Slenker N, Ratigan B. The Association of a Varus Hindfoot and Fracture of the Fifth Metatarsal Metaphyseal-Diaphyseal Junction: The Jones fracture. Am J Sports Med 2008;36(7):1367–72.

46. Fetzer GB, Wright RW. Metatarsal Shaft Fractures and Fractures of the Proximal Fifth Metatarsal. Clin Sports Med 2006;25:139–50.

47. Attia AK, Taha T, Kong G, et al. Return to Play and Fracture Union After the Surgical Management of Jones Fractures in Athletes: A systematic review and meta-analysis. Am J Sports Med 2021;49(12):3422–36.

48. O'Malley M, Desandis B, Allen A, et al. Operative Treatment of Fifth Metatarsal Jones Fractures (Zones II and III) in the NBA. Foot Ankle Int 2016;37(5):488–500.

49. Kavanaugh JH, Brower TD, Mann RV. The Jones Fracture Revisited. J Bone Joint Surg 1978;60:776–82.

50. Simkin A, Leichter J, Giladi M, et al. Combined Effect of Foot Arch Structure and an Orthotic Device on Stress Fractures. Foot Ankle 1989;10(1):25–9.

51. Lee KT, Kim KC, Park YU, et al. Radiographic Evaluation of Foot Structure Following Fifth Metatarsal Stress Fracture. Foot Ankle Int 2011;32(8):796–801.

52. Carreira DS, Sandilands SM. Radiographic Factors and Effect of Fifth Metatarsal Jones and Diaphyseal Stress Fractures on Participation in the NFL. Foot Ankle Int 2013;34(4):518–22.

53. Spang RC, Haber DB, Beaulieu-Jones BR, et al. Jones Fractures Identified at the National Football League Scouting Combine: Assessment of prognostic factors, computed tomography findings, and initial career performance. Orthop J Sports Med 2018;6(8). 2325967118790740.

54. Granata JD, Berlet GC, Philbin TM, et al. Failed Surgical Management of Acute Proximal Fifth Metatarsal (Jones) Fractures: A retrospective case series and literature review. Foot Ankle Spec 2015;8:454–9.

55. Jones CP. Cavovarus. Clin Sports Med 2020;39(4):793–9.
56. Hunt KJ, Anderson RB. Treatment of Jones Fracture Nonunions and Refractures in the Elite Athlete. Am J Sports Med 2011;39(9):1948–54.
57. Karlsson J, Eriksson BI, Bergsten T, et al. Comparison of Two Anatomic Reconstructions for Chronic Lateral instability of the Ankle Joint. Am J Sports Med 1997;25(1):48–53.
58. Keller M, Grossman J, Caron M, et al. Lateral ankle instability and the Brostrom-Gould procedure. J Foot Ankle Surg 1996;35(6):513–20.
59. Irwin TA. Techniques for Cavovarus Foot Reconstruction with Concomitant Ankle Instability. Operat Tech Orthop 2022;32(3):100985.
60. Easley ME, Latt DL, Santangelo JR, et al. Osteochondral Lesions of the Talus. Am Acad Orthop Surg 2010;18(10):616–30.
61. Becher C, Thermann H. Results of Microfracture in the Treatment of Articular Cartilage Defects of the Talus. Foot Ankle Int 2005;26(8):583–9.
62. Adams SB, Viens NA, Easley ME, et al. Midterm Results of Osteochondral Lesions of the Talar Shoulder Treated with Fresh Osteochondral Allograft Transplantation. J Bone Joint Surg 2011;93(7):648–54.
63. Easley ME, Vineyard JC. Varus Ankle and Osteochondral Lesions of the Talus. Foot Ankle Clin 2012;17(1):21–38.
64. Hunter LJ, Fortune J. Foot and ankle biomechanics. S Afr J Physiother 2000; 56(1):17–20.
65. Malahias MA, Cantiller EB, Kadu VV, et al. The Clinical Outcome of Endoscopic Plantar Fascia Release: A current concept review. Foot Ankle Surg 2020;26(1): 19–24.
66. Shamrock AG, Varacallo M., (2019) Achilles Tendon Ruptures. Nih.gov. Available at: https://www.ncbi.nlm.nih.gov/books/NBK430844/.
67. Carmont MR. Achilles Tendon Rupture: The evaluation and outcome of percutaneous and minimally invasive repair. Br J Sports Med 2018;52(19):1281–2.
68. Zou Y, Li X, Wang L, et al. Endoscopically Assisted, Minimally Invasive Reconstruction for Chronic Achilles Tendon Rupture With a Double-Bundle Flexor Hallucis Longus. Orthopaedic Journal of Sports Medicine 2021;9(3). 232596712097999.
69. Lui TH. Endoscopic Management of Recalcitrant Retrofibular Pain Without Peroneal Tendon Subluxation or Dislocation. Arch Orthop Trauma Surg 2011;132(3): 357–61.
70. Nishikawa DRC, Duarte FA, Saito GH, et al. Minimally Invasive Tenodesis for Peroneus Longus Tendon Rupture: A case report and review of literature. World J Orthoped 2020;11(2):137–44.
71. Stiglitz Y, Cazeau C. Minimally Invasive Surgery and Percutaneous Surgery of the Hindfoot and Midfoot. Eur J Orthop Surg Traumatol 2018;28(5):839–47.
72. Perez-Carro L, Rodrigo-Arriaza C, Trueba-Sanchez L, et al. Arthroscopic-Assisted Arthrodesis in the Foot and Ankle. Subtalar, Tibiotalar, Tibiocalcaneal, and Metatarsophalangeal: 25 years of experience. J Arthrosc Surg Sports Med 2021;2(2):87–93.
73. Panchbhavi VK. Percutaneous Techniques for Tendon Transfers in the Foot and Ankle. Foot Ankle Clin 2014;19(1):113–22.

Toes Deformities in Cavovarus
How to Approach Them

Barbara Piclet-Legré, MD[a], Véronique Darcel, MD[b],*

KEYWORDS

- Cavus foot • Lesser toe deformities • Tendon transfer • Tenotomies
- Osteotomy arthrodesis • Percutaneous surgery

KEY POINTS

- Surgery is performed when conservative measures fails. Therapeutic choices are made from proximal to distal, and surgical management of toe deformities in pes cavus is only considered after treatment of the symptomatic overlying deformities.
- Joint sparing procedure as flexor to extensor transfer or percutaneous procedures including tenotomies, arthrolysis, and osteotomies are indicated for the treatment of reducible LTD.
- Arthrodesis or arthroplasties are the best option for rigid LTD in association with tendon transfer or percutaneous procedures depending of surgeon's experience and patient's clinical examination.

INTRODUCTION

Lesser toe deformities (LTD) in cavus foot can take all forms but the sagittal ones are the most frequent. They are painful and require an etiological screening to identify any underlying neurological disease such as Charcot Marie Tooth (CMT) disease. Their management are challenging based on a combination of osseous and soft tissue procedures to restore muscular balance.

The aim of the present study was to provide an update on classification and surgical management of LTD in cavus foot including percutaneous procedures with a special focus on sagittal deformities.

SAGITTAL DEFORMITIES PATHOPHYSIOLOGY

Muscle imbalance is the key of cavovarus foot type development.[1]

[a] Department of Orthopaedics, Centre du pied, La Ciotat, Marseille, France; [b] Department of Orthopaedics, Maison de Santé Protestante de Bordeaux Bagatelle, Bordeaux, France
* Corresponding author.
E-mail address: v.darcel@mspb.com

Foot Ankle Clin N Am 28 (2023) 743–757
https://doi.org/10.1016/j.fcl.2023.06.005
1083-7515/23/© 2023 Elsevier Inc. All rights reserved.

foot.theclinics.com

Cavovarus foot in CMT is a model of muscle imbalance: the neuropathy weakens tibialis anterior and peroneus brevis. Unopposed action of tibialis posterior and peroneus longus leads to plantar flexion of the first ray, which increases the hindfoot varus.[1]

Intrinsic muscles (interosseous and lumbrical) paralysis or paresis leads to a biomechanical advantage of the extrinsic muscles.

Sagittal lesser toes deformities mainly result from imbalance between the intrinsic and extrinsic muscles of the foot or from capsule-ligament stabilizer failure by mechanical overloading of the joints.[2,3] Chronic metatarso-phalangeal joint (MTP) hyperextension progressively induces stretching then failure of the plantar stabilizers, worsening the intrinsic muscles ineffective and causing muscle imbalance in favor of flexion.

As a reminder, the extensor tendons have no action powerful than on the proximal phalanx (P1) by the effect "strap" of the fibro-aponeurotic hood, and the flexor tendons act only on the phalanges intermediate and distal (P2 and P3); balance is not restored only by the interosseous and lumbrical muscles. In a word, MTP joints are extended by extrinsic and flexed by intrinsic and it is the other way around for IP joints.

TOES DEFORMITIES ANALYSIS

In adults, the most common reason for consultation is a conflict with the shoe related to sagittal toes deformities, a pulp overpressure, or metatarsalgia. Careful clinical examination is essential to successful management of LTD in pes cavus, especially in subtle cavovarus. Evaluation of the entire body is mandatory with complete neurological, muscle and joints examination.

Etiological Assessment is Essential

Cavus foot is a common symptom of very different pathologies (**Table 1**) and can be indicative of a neurological impairment such as hereditary motor and sensory neuropathies (HMSN) including Charcot Mary Tooth (CMT) disease.[4–8]

Posttraumatic causes are less frequent.

Idiopathic or subtle cavus foot is a mild misalignment diagnoses by elimination, and it has no neurophysiological difference with healthy population but could have some symptoms of clinical impairment.[9,10]

Functional Impact of Lateral Toe Deformities and Clinical Examination

The main reason for consultation will guide the observation of the weight-bearing posture of the foot and the footwear.

Deformity analysis

Deformity analysis is guided by a precise and standardized morphologic description and systematic classification of lesser toe deformity (LTD) proposed in 2013 by Dr Piclet, at the Association Française de Chirurgie du Pied (AFCP) congress in Lille then modified in collaboration with the AFCP.[11]

It describes the position of each toe-joint, from proximal to distal, in terms of the position of the distal segment with respect to its anatomic position. Each lesser toe is referenced by its number (2–5) and 3 letters, 1 per joint. In the sagittal plane, the position of the distal segment is coded "f" for flexion, "n" for neutral or "e" for extension (**Fig. 1**). When there is no sagittal deformity (distal segment of joint in neutral position [n]), the deformation in the horizontal plane can be considered and denoted "m" when the distal segment is deviated in medial and "l" when it is deviated in lateral (**Fig. 2**). This is the only classification in which intraobserver and interobserver reproducibility has been assessed for second toe deformity.[11] However, it does not provide information about reducibility, toe ground contact, joint stability, or radiologic characteristics.

Table 1
Summary table of the main causes of pes cavus

Neurological	Traumatic	Clubfoot	Others
• HMSN,	• Compartment	• Untreated	• Idiopathic
• Cerebral palsy	syndrome	• Undertreated	• Tarsal coalition
• Stroke sequelae	• Talar neck malunion		• Rheumatoid arthritis
• Anterior horn disease	• Peroneal nerve injury		• Ankle osteoarthritis
• Spinal cord lesions	• Knee dislocation		• Plantar fibromatosis
• Poliomyelitis	• Scar tissue		• Varus subtalar joint
• Myelomeningocele	• Burns		axis
• Polyneuritic	• Vascular lesions		• Diabetic foot
syndromes	• Hindfoot instability		syndrome
• Parkinson disease	• Tibial fractures		
• Huntington chorea	• Calcaneal malunion		
• Friedreich ataxia,			
amyotrophic lateral			
sclerosis			
• leprosy			
• Roussy-Levy			
syndrome			
• Stumpell-Lorrain			
disease			
• Pierre-Marie			
heredotaxy			

Reducibility analysis

In non–weight-bearing, the reducibility of each joint is tested with a passive mobilization of the affected joint and with the push-up test pressing under the metatarsal head. The terms used are flexible (f), semirigid (sr), or rigid (r).

After traumatic injury as a posterior compartment syndroma by flexor digitorum longus (FDL) and FHL contracture, deformity appears or worsens in ankle dorsal flexion and disappears in ankle plantar flexion.[12]

Metatarso-phalangeal joint instability

Patients usually complain of joint pain, intensified underweight-bearing, associated with malalignment of the toe.

At the synovitis stage, the "V" sign is the first seen on clinical examination. In charge, barefoot, it happens an abnormal gap between the affected toe and its neighbor.[13]

The clinical evaluation of the plantar plate (PP) is done by palpating the MTP and using the drawer test.[14]

Toe ground contact

Toe ground contact quality is assessed in weight-bearing by the paper pull-out test (ability to keep a sheet of paper on the ground using toe pressure against pull-out) or on the French Foot Surgery Association (AFCP) podoscopic toe ground contact area classification, with scores for active and passive pressure in each toe[15]: score 0 for passive toe ground contact increase when active, score 1 for only active toe ground contact, and score 2 when there is no contact, neither active nor passive.

Associated Causes of Mechanical Overload in the Forefoot

Whether in subtle or severe cavus foot, mechanical overload in the forefoot may be increased by an equinus, a gastrocnemius tightness, which is systematically searched for with the Silfverskïold test, and a mechanical forefoot deformity as a bunion.

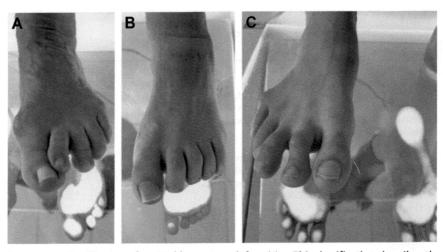

Fig. 1. AFCP classification of sagittal lesser toes deformities. This classification describes the position of each segment of the toe from proximal to distal taking into account in the first place the sagittal deformation, the position of the MTP is denoted "e" when the proximal phalanx is in extension, "n" when it is in neutral position and "f" when in flexion. We proceed in the same way for the PIP and the DIP. AFCP: French association of foot surgery. (*A*): 2efn is the most frequent in subtle PC. (*B*): 2eff is more usual if there is a neurological etiology. This case shows also a 3nfn. (*C*): 2efe is rare.

Complementary Examination About Lateral Toe Deformities

X-ray shows and quantifies the deformities, assesses MTP subluxation or dislocation, and sheds light on associated causes (pes cavus, hallux valgus, metatarsal head erosion, osteoarthritis, brachymetatarsia, and so forth).

Ultrasound demonstrates synovitis and studies the PP.[16]

MRI shows 95% sensitivity and 100% specificity in diagnosing PP lesions.[17]

Neurological investigations are best performed by a neurologist including electro-diagnostic studies if necessary.

TREATMENTS
Nonoperative Management

Nonsurgical treatment of toe deformities in cavus foot includes a footwear adaptation with a high and large toe box. Custom-made orthoses are efficient in reducing chronic musculoskeletal foot pain associated with pes cavus.[18] An insole with retro-capital or bar support is advised for patient with flexible sagittal toe deformities. In case of fixed deformity of the toes, stabilizing orthoses are preferred to corrective orthoses. Corrective toe braces for reducible deformities or protective braces for irreducible deformities, tube bandages, and corrective strappings and tapings reduce frictions pain.[19] For severe and rigid LTD, custom-made shoes are required.

Gastrocnemius stretching program is associated in case of associated equinus when the Silfverskiöld test is positive. A 12 weeks, program increased ankle range of motion and functional outcomes for children with CMT.[20]

Intramuscular botulinum toxin injections have been tested to prevent pes cavus progression in children with Charcot-Marie-Tooth disease type1A (CMTA1) in a 24-month follow-up, randomized single blind study. Tolerance and safety was proved but injections did not affect the progression of cavus foot.[21]

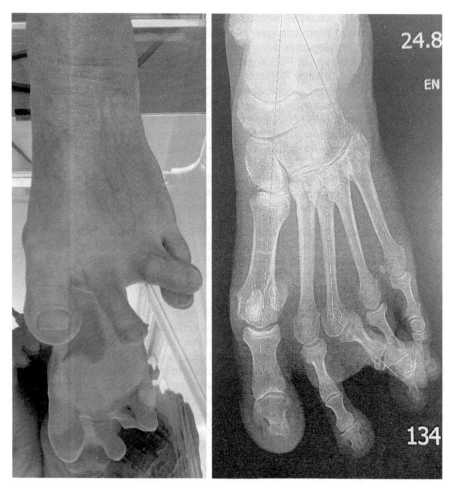

Fig. 2. *AFCP classification of horizontal lesser toes deformities.* 3lff with MTP3 subluxation.

Surgical Treatment

The surgical treatment is considered if there is insufficient relief with optimal nonsurgical management. The objective is to reduce pain and improve walking and footwear. A wide variety of procedures for the treatment of LTD has been described involving soft tissue procedures and bony procedures including osteotomies and arthrodesis.

Soft tissue procedures

Tendon lengthening and tenotomies. Open or percutaneous lengthening of the overall Achilles tendon or only of the gastrocnemius by the Barouk or Stryer technique[22] depends on the result of the Silfverskiöld test.

Extensor or flexor forefoot tenotomies can be open or percutaneous and are often associated with arthrolysis, osteotomies, or arthrodesis. Extensor lengthening or tenotomy is used for deformities with the MTP in dorsal flexion. Percutaneously, a paratendon approach is required adjacent to the MTP joint. Dorsal MTP arthrolysis may be associated.[23,24]

Flexor digitorum brevis (FDB) tenotomy is associated to P1 osteotomy for reducible deformity in proximal interphalangeal joint (PIP) flexion.[23] The approach is medial or lateral depending on surgeon's dominant hand and right or left foot. The toe is held in flexion while 2 P1 slips of FDB are percutaneously released by rotating a beaver against the condyles. Plantar PIP arthrolysis is performed simultaneously.[23] Isolated FDB tenotomy via the plantar approach at the base of P1 has been described[24] where the FDB is superficial but there is a higher risk of not being selective.

Tenotomy or lengthening of FDL is used for reducible distal interphalangeal joint (DIP) deformity in plantar flexion. DIP plantar release is always associated. It uses a plantar approach centered below the DIP, or a medial or a lateral approach similar to PIP approach.

Tenotomy of both flexors can be performed for reducible deformity in PIP and DIP flexion by a plantar approach centered below the MTP joint.[24] The effectiveness is judged by a maneuver in dorsal flexion of the toe simultaneously.

Arthrolysis. Dorsal percutaneous or open MTP dorsal release is often necessary in addition to extensors lengthening or tenotomies for the treatment of flexible toe deformities with MTP extension. Similarly, PIP or DIP release is associated with FDB or FDL percutaneous tenotomies for flexible deformities with PIP or DIP flexion.[23,24]

Tendon transfers

Jones procedure Described by Sir Robert Jones in 1916 for the treatment of clawfoot coexisting with a claw hallux. [25,26] The claw hallux or cook up deformity is defined as an extension of the MTP joint and a flexion of interphalangeal joint (IPJ) of the hallux. Jones procedure consists of the transfer of the distal part of the extensor hallux longus through the neck of the first metatarsal from lateral to medial, which is tied on itself at the dorsal part of the metatarsal. The IPJ fusion of the hallux was added to the original description in recent literature for the treatment of rigid deformity as modified Jones procedure. The study of Breusch and colleagues[27] evaluated retrospectively the results of 81 Jones modified procedures. The rate of satisfaction was 86% and malposition of the toe was corrected in 80 feet (**Fig. 3**).

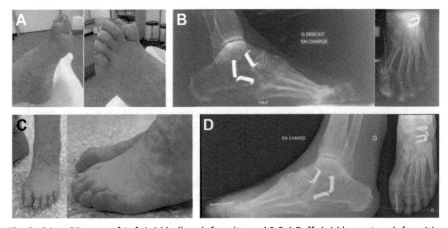

Fig. 3. 3A et 3B: case of 1ef rigid hallux deformity and 2,3,4,5eff rigid lesser toe deformities postpoliomyelitis with clinical (A) and radiological aspect (B). 3C et 3D: after surgical treatment of hallux deformity by Jones procedure and lesser toe deformities by extensors percutaneous tenotomies and PIP fusions using a radiotransparent implant (second and third toes) and arthroplasties (fourth and fifth toes): clinical (C) and radiological (D) results.

FDL transfer (Girdlestone-Taylor) This procedure can be used alone for flexible deformities with MTP in extension and PIP and DIP in flexion, and in association with a PIP arthrodesis for rigid deformities. It was popularized by Girdlestone and Taylor and was later published with many variations.[28,29] FDL is detached from its distal insertion below the DIP and then splited into 2 sleeps, which are passed on either side of the proximal phalanx (P1). Then, it is sutured to the extensor hood. Losa-Iglesia and colleagues[30] found good satisfaction result in their meta-analysis after FDL transfer for the treatment of LTD.

Tenodesis variants were described: passing the FDL through a transosseous tunnel from plantar to dorsal at the P1 base and fixing it with an interference screw, or fixing it to the plantar side of P1 with an anchor or tenodesis screw.[31]

FDB transfer (Pisani) In the same way, FDB can be used alone for surgical treatment of flexible LTD with MTP in extension and PIP in flexion and in association with a PIP fusion or arthroplasty when the deformity is rigid. The 2 distal slips of the FDB are detached from the PIP and are passed on either side of P1 and then sutured to the extensor hood.[32] The tendon is smaller than FDL, which makes it trickier to manage. Therefore, it is rarely used for pes cavus (PC).

FDB transfer to FDL This transfer was designed for the management of LTD after traumatic injury without intrinsic muscle palsy. This deformity usually occurs after posterior compartment syndroma by FDL and FHL contracture. In this case, deformity appears or worsens in ankle dorsal flexion and disappears in ankle plantar flexion. The transfer consists in FDL tenotomy at the MTP and suture of the distal stump onto the distal stump of the FDB released from P1.[12,31] Gonçalves and colleagues[12] found a restauration of toe flexion and esthetic aspect of 10 of 10 affected patients after this transfer.

EDL transfer (Hibbs procedure) Hibbs tenosuspension is used alone for reducible deformities due to extensor recruitment and in association with a PIP arthrodesis for semireducible or fixed LTD.[33,34] The typical indication is patient with a weak dorsiflexion of the foot and varus at the swing phase with LTD, what can happen in the CMT or postpolio syndrome. The extensor digitorum longus (EDL) is transferred to the peroneus tertius or to the cuboid to assist with dorsal flexion and eversion of the foot. The distal slips of EDL tendons are transferred to the corresponding transected extensor digitorum brevis (EDB) tendons proximal to the MTP joint. The same principal and surgical technique could be used for the management of reducible cook up deformity of the hallux in the article of DiDomenico and colleagues.[34]

Bony procedures

Open and percutaneous unicortical or bicortical osteotomies of phalanxes. They are described for flexible toe deformities. P1 osteotomy is best located in the metaphyseal part proximal to P1 to optimize union time. It can be performed using the same plantar approach used for the tenotomy of both flexors, approaching the bone slightly laterally relative to the flexor tendons unless a complete tenotomy was decided, which is rare in our surgical practice. An oblique phalangeal osteotomy has been described by Michel Bénichou, which increases shortening effect. In our practice, P1 oblique osteotomy is often performed using the lateral plantar approach for selective FDB tenotomy, making both gestures with one way (**Fig. 4**). This oblique P1 osteotomy, not necessarily with the aim to shorten, gives larger contact surfaces that improve the stabilization and probably also bone consolidation.

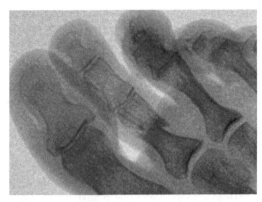

Fig. 4. Percutaneous oblique P1 osteotomy.

P2 osteotomy is middiaphyseal to avoid break-in articular and is performed by a lateral or medial approach depending on surgeon's dominant hand and right or left foot. Unicortical, it allows a flexion or extension effect in sagittal plane and a varisation or a valgisation effect in axial plane. Bicortical, it allows a shortening or a rotation of the intermediate phalanx.

Osteotomies are performed in association with tendon lengthening or tenotomies and joint release most of the time.[23] Lesser toes are maintained in intrinsic plus position for 6 weeks after surgery using a postoperative bandage or a K-wire fixation.

Proximal interphalangeal joint or distal interphalangeal joint arthrodesis or arthroplasties. They are used to treat rigid deformities.[1] End-to-end fusion requires a fixation. Traditionally, a Kirshner-wire was recommended. More recently, several intramedullary fixation devices have been developed with various composition and design.[35] The systematic review of Mirmiran and Younger about lesser digits implants concludes that all categories of fixation methods can be considered if used appropriately, considering surgeon's experience and patient's clinical examination and personal goal.[35] Other surgical techniques as peg in hole procedure are published.[36]

OPERATIVE TREATMENTS INDICATION

Cavovarus surgery is considered if medical treatment fails to control the symptoms.

The objective is to reduce pain and improve walking and footwear. The surgeon must consider the cause of the deformation, its location, its reducibility or its rigidity, and the muscular balance.

Because correction of the midfoot can improve flexible forefoot deformities, usually toe surgery is programmed at the end of PC surgery.

Therapeutic choices are made from proximal to distal, and surgical management of toe deformities in pes cavus is only considered after treatment of the symptomatic overlying deformities.

The attitude varies according to the presence of a neurological cause.

Without Neurological Impairment: Subtle Cavus Foot (Idiopathic Cavus Deformity)

Percutaneous approach strategy is proximal to distal according to AFCP classification with sequential correction addressing MTP deformity before going on to the PIP and DIP. Reducibility and surgeon's habits will make the surgery "à la carte" allowing the association of percutaneous and open gestures.

For metatarso-phalangeal joint dorsiflexion deformity (classified enn, efn, eff in Association Française de Chirurgie du Pied classification)

One can choose a percutaneous extensor tenotomy or an open lengthening with a Z-plasty. Ideally, the percutaneous tenotomy is performed in the area where the 2 tendons (EDB and EDL) are well individualized, adjacent to the MTP joint. The success criterion is often visual in CF with visible tendons (**Fig. 5**).

A dorsal MTP release can be added if necessary. It is the logical extension in depth extensor tenotomy but sometimes the latter are offset laterally. A pull on the toe allows the joint to be uncoupled in order to facilitate the entry of the beaver blade in certain dislocated toes cases.

Any associated proximal interphalangeal joint or distal interphalangeal joint deformity

It will be corrected after MTP correction.

Selective percutaneous flexor tenotomies can be used alone or more often associated to bone or joint procedures.

FDB tenotomy is associated to P1 osteotomy for reducible deformity in PIP flexion. FDB tenotomy is not always necessary in a PIP deformity, especially when a shortening possible of P1 allows to relax the shortened tendons.

FDL tenotomy can be done for reducible DIP deformity in plantar flexion.

P1 osteotomy is more often bicortical for convenience but also by necessity, it can be shortened in case of deformation old stiffened with a tendon relaxation effect or if the toe is too long. In monocortical one, the surgeon can obtain a plantar flexion or the correction of an horizontal toe deviation.

P2 osteotomy can be a useful complement when PIP flexion correction is not enough with FDB tenotomy, PIP release and P1 osteotomy. Monocortical at best, P2 osteotomy allows correction of a horizontal deviation of the DIP or sometimes a dorsal flexion. Bicortical, it allows a shortening of the intermediate phalanx but with a risk of postoperative edema that can be reduced using temporary percutaneous pinning avoiding any movement in the osteotomy.

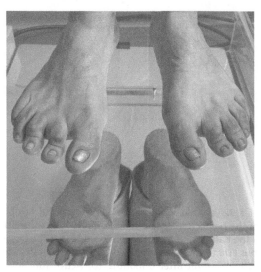

Fig. 5. PC with visible extensor tendons allowing visual criteria success for tenotomies adjacent to the MTP joint.

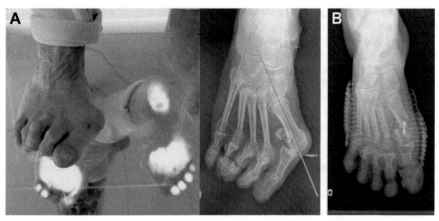

Fig. 6. (*A*) A case of a 78-year-old woman painful semirigid 234 efn (according to AFCP classification) and severe bunion making shoes wearing almost impossible. Radiograph shows MTP dislocation of less than 5mm on second and third rays. (*B*) We performed percutaneous selective tenotomies of second and third LTD (extensors and FDB), P1 osteotomies for second, third, and fourth LTD, MTP 2-3 release, DMMO 2-3 and MIS bunion osteotomies.

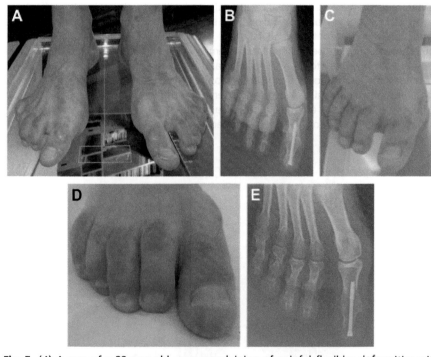

Fig. 7. (*A*) A case of a 32-year-old man complaining of painful flexibles deformities with cock up deformity of the hallux and 2345 efn (according to AFCP classification). (*B*) We performed IPJ fusion of the hallux, and percutaneous gestures for the lesser toes: extensor and selective percutaneous FDB tenotomies with P1 osteotomies plus P2 osteotomies for second and third toes. (*C*) Clinical result after 6 months. (*D*) Active function after percutaneous extensor and FDB tenotomies for LTD. (*E*) Radiological aspect after 6 months with an incomplete fusion of P1 osteotomy of the fourth toe without symptoms.

We have studied the effectiveness of percutaneous gestures since more than 10 years. Our publication in Orthopedics and traumatology: surgery and research in 2015 enabled us to present a prospective series of 57 cases of PIP deformity of the second toe (AFCP nfn or efn).[23] We excluded from this study any metatarsal osteotomy in order to judge the result of the toes targeted gestures. After 2 years, we got an identical patient and surgeon satisfaction almost 90% concerning the correction of the PIP deformity and active plantar flexion of the toe.

Métatarsal osteotomies in cavo varus foot

Percutaneous surgery is a real progress for MTP instability[37,38] in our practices but indication of metatarsal osteotomies is subtle in cavo varus foot.

We must always remember the risk of transfer metatarsalgia particularly on the first and the fifth rays with percutaneous neck metatarsal osteotomies distal metatarsal metaphysal osteotomy (DMMO).

In our practice, in subtle PC, we perform DMMO limited to the second and third metatarsals as a reliable solution in the management of metatarsalgia by lesion of the PP associated with hallux valgus. We presented in AFCP spring meeting in Barcelona 2022 a retrospective single-operator study of 118 feet: the risk of transfer metatarsalgia was not increased compared with the data of literature (**Fig. 6**).

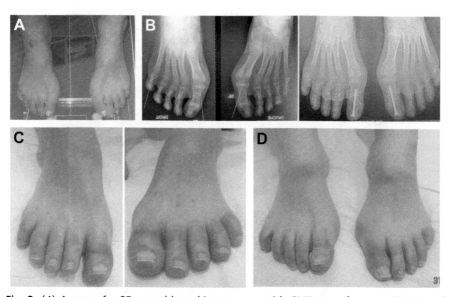

Fig. 8. (*A*) A case of a 25-year-old smoking woman with CMT cavus foot complaining of painful semirigid LTD and rigid cock up deformity making it difficult to wear foot orthotics in shoes. (*B*). We decided together to realize IPJ fusion of the hallux for both hallux deformities but different technics for LTD in each foot. On the left foot conventional technics with Girdlestone transfer and PIP fusion for 234 eff according to AFCP classification and resection arthroplasty of the fifth toe; percutaneous extensor tenotomies were associated. The right foot LDT was corrected with extensor and selective percutaneous FDL tenotomies with P1 osteotomies. (*C*). The immediate postoperative follow-up was easier for her in the conventional technics operated foot probably because of the pinning immobilizing the corrected toes and the inconvenience of rigorous dressings for the percutaneous foot. (*D*). Long-term result improved her comfort with an identical result for LTD correction but also for stiffness!

Conventional technics are decided for severe dislocations and according cases.

What about conventional surgical technics?

Percutaneous gestures can be associated with conventional technics as tools.

Either in the same toe for noncompliant patients for which we can combine a temporary DIP and/or PIP pinning with percutaneous gestures or association of percutaneous tenotomies and PIP or DIP fusion for rigid toes.

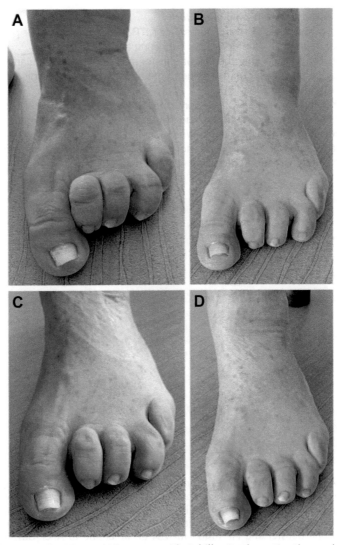

Fig. 9. (*A*) A case of a 76-year-old woman with Achilles tendon retraction and complaints about metatarsalgia and flexible eff deformities according to AFCP classification. (*B*) We first did a Strayer and a retromalleolar open lengthening of the FDL, which relieved metatarsalgia and improved LTD after 45 days. (*C*) One year after she still complained about 2efn and 3efn (according to AFCP classification): we used percutaneous gestures (extensors and FDB tenotomies) associated with conventional technics (PIP fusion). (*D*) Five months later, she was really improved to wear shoes.

Different technics may be decided for each toe: Jones procedure with IPJ fusion of the hallux,[39] PIP resection arthroplasty of the fifth toe, and so many imaginable combinations with percutaneous surgery (**Fig. 7**).

Achilles tendon lengthening or isolated gastrocnemius recession (Strayer or Barouk technique) is sometimes necessary in association.[22]

In posttraumatic injuries, with extrinsic flexors shortness as after posterior compartment syndrome of the leg, a FDB transfer to FDL described by Valtin is indicated.[12]

With Neurological Impairment

For flexible deformities, flexor to extensor tendon transfers (Girdlestone transfer) may be performed to improve the realignment of the toes after midfoot correction.[34] Hibbs tenosuspension is useful for reducible LTD with recruitment of EDL due to tibialis anterior tendon weakness.

In case of rigid deformities, those procedures can be used in association with a PIP fusion.

Percutaneous phalangeal osteotomies seem to have few drawbacks particularly for stiffness results (**Fig. 8**). The advantages of percutaneous gestures regards the operative time, which is twice as fast and skin scarring. Disadvantages are the inconvenience of rigorous dressings, which can be more painful compared with pinning immobilization. That is why we prefer conventional care for both the surgeon and the patient.

Tenotomy of both flexors is sometimes sufficient for neurological deformities (AFCP nff) (**Fig. 9**).

Spastic cases are best decided by a neurologist for neurotomies.

CLINICS CARE POINTS

- Sagittal LTD is the most common in cavus foot. They mainly result from imbalance between the intrinsic and extrinsic muscles of the foot.

- They require an etiological screening to identify any underlying neurological disease such as CMT disease.

- Analysis of the deformity considers its cause, its morphological classification, its reducibility or irreducibility and the stability of the métatarso-phalangeal joint.

- Surgery is performed when conservative measures fails. Therapeutic choices are made from proximal to distal, and surgical management of toe deformities in pes cavus is only considered after treatment of the symptomatic overlying deformities.

- Joint sparing procedure as flexor to extensor transfer or percutaneous procedures including tenotomies, arthrolysis, and osteotomies are indicated for the treatment of reducible LTD.

- Arthrodesis or arthroplasties are the best option for rigid LTD in association with tendon transfer or percutaneous procedures depending of surgeon's experience and patient's clinical examination.

DISCLOSURE

V. Darcel: consulting (FH orthopedics et General electrics); B. Piclet-Legré: Royalties Euros, Roman industry.

REFERENCES

1. Krause FG, Wing KJ, Younger ASE. Neuromuscular issues in cavovarus foot. Foot Ankle Clin 2008;13(2):243–58, vi.

2. Barg A, Courville XF, Nickisch F, et al. Role of collateral ligaments in metatarso-phalangeal stability: a cadaver study. Foot Ankle Int 2012;33(10):877–82.

3. Chalayon O, Chertman C, Guss AD, et al. Role of plantar plate and surgical reconstruction techniques on static stability of lesser metatarsophalangeal joints: a biomechanical study. Foot Ankle Int 2013;34(10):1436–42.

4. Seaman TJ, Ball TA. Pes Cavus. In: StatPearls. StatPearls Publishing; 2023. Available at: http://www.ncbi.nlm.nih.gov/books/NBK556016/. Accessed May 24, 2023.

5. Younger ASE, Hansen ST. Adult cavovarus foot. J Am Acad Orthop Surg 2005; 13(5):302–15.

6. Krähenbühl N, Weinberg MW. Anatomy and biomechanics of cavovarus deformity. Foot Ankle Clin 2019;24(2):173–81.

7. Rosenbaum AJ, Lisella J, Patel N, et al. The cavus foot. Med Clin North Am 2014; 98(2):301–12.

8. Piazza S, Ricci G, Caldarazzo Ienco E, et al. Pes cavus and hereditary neuropathies: when a relationship should be suspected. J Orthop Traumatol 2010;11(4): 195–201.

9. Di Fabio R, Lispi L, Santorelli FM, et al. Idiopathic pes cavus in adults is not associated with neurophysiological impairment in the lower limbs. Neurol Sci 2015; 36(12):2287–90.

10. Deben SE, Pomeroy GC. Subtle cavus foot: diagnosis and management. J Am Acad Orthop Surg 2014;22(8):512–20.

11. Lintz F, Beldame J, Kerhousse G, et al. Intra- and inter-observer reliability of the AFCP classification for sagittal plane deformities of the second toe. Foot Ankle Surg 2020;26(6):650–6.

12. Gonçalves H, Kajetanek C, Graff W, et al. Flexor digitorum brevis tendon transfer to the flexor digitorum longus tendon according to Valtin in posttraumatic flexible claw toe deformity due to extrinsic toe flexor shortening. Orthop Traumatol Surg Res 2015;101(2):257–60.

13. Panchbhavi VK, Trevino S. Clinical tip: a new clinical sign associated with metatarsophalangeal joint synovitis of the lesser toes. Foot Ankle Int 2007;28(5):640–1.

14. Coughlin MJ, Baumfeld DS, Nery C. Second MTP joint instability: grading of the deformity and description of surgical repair of capsular insufficiency. Phys Sportsmed 2011;39(3):132–41.

15. Bernasconi A, Beldame J, Darcel V, et al. Podoscopic classification of second toe deformities. Foot Ankle Surg 2021;27(7):750–4.

16. McCarthy CL, Thompson GV. Ultrasound findings of plantar plate tears of the lesser metatarsophalangeal joints. Skeletal Radiol 2021;50(8):1513–25.

17. Sung W, Weil L, Weil LS, et al. Diagnosis of plantar plate injury by magnetic resonance imaging with reference to intraoperative findings. J Foot Ankle Surg 2012; 51(5):570–4.

18. Burns J, Crosbie J, Ouvrier R, et al. Effective orthotic therapy for the painful cavus foot: a randomized controlled trial. J Am Podiatr Med Assoc 2006;96(3):205–11.

19. Federer AE, Tainter DM, Adams SB, et al. Conservative management of metatarsalgia and lesser toe deformities. Foot Ankle Clin 2018;23(1):9–20.

20. Burns J, Raymond J, Ouvrier R. Feasibility of foot and ankle strength training in childhood charcot-marie-tooth disease. Neuromuscul Disord NMD 2009;19(12): 818–21.

21. Burns J, Scheinberg A, Ryan MM, et al. Randomized trial of botulinum toxin to prevent pes cavus progression in pediatric Charcot-Marie-Tooth disease type 1A. Muscle Nerve 2010;42(2):262–7.

22. Hsu RY, VanValkenburg S, Tanriover A, et al. Surgical techniques of gastrocnemius lengthening. Foot Ankle Clin 2014;19(4):745–65.
23. Frey-Ollivier S, Catena F, Hélix-Giordanino M, et al. Treatment of flexible lesser toe deformities. Foot Ankle Clin 2018;23(1):69–90.
24. Prado MD, Ripoll PL, Golanó P. Cirugía percutánea del pie. Técnicas quirúrgicas. Indicaciones. Bases anatómicas | Revista Española de Cirugía Ortopédica y TraumatologíaCirugía percutánea del pie: técnicas quirúrgicas, indicaciones. Elsevier; 2003.
25. Derner R, Holmes J. Jones tendon transfer. Clin Podiatr Med Surg 2016;33(1): 55–62.
26. Jones R III. The soldier's foot and the treatment of common deformities of the foot. Br Med J 1916;1(2891):749–53.
27. Breusch SJ, Wenz W, Döderlein L. Function after correction of a clawed great toe by a modified Robert Jones transfer. J Bone Joint Surg Br 2000;82(2):250–4.
28. Girdlestone GR. Physiotherapy for hand and foot. Physiotherapy 1947;32(11): 167–9.
29. Cove R, Cooke PH, Thomason K. The Oxford procedure for the treatment of lesser toe deformities. Ann R Coll Surg Engl 2011;93(7):553–4.
30. Losa Iglesias ME, Becerro de Bengoa Vallejo R, Jules KT, et al. Meta-analysis of flexor tendon transfer for the correction of lesser toe deformities. J Am Podiatr Med Assoc 2012;102(5):359–68.
31. Valtin B, Leemrijse T. Pathologie des orteils: clinique et traitement chirurgical. In: Pathologie Du Pied et de La Cheville. Tsunami. Masson; :227-242.
32. Leemrijse T., Valtin B., Trasposizione del flessore superficiale di II-III-IV-V dito alla falange basale pro interossei - Chirurgia del Piede 2009 December;33(3):161-162. Available at: https://www.minervamedica.it/it/riviste/chirurgia-piede/articolo. php?cod=R32Y2009N03A0161 Accessed October 31, 2021.
33. Grambart ST. Hibbs Tenosuspension. Clin Podiatr Med Surg 2016;33(1):63–9.
34. DiDomenico LA, Rizkalla J, Cartman J, et al. Hallux and lesser digits deformities associated with cavus foot. Clin Podiatr Med Surg 2021;38(3):343–60.
35. Mirmiran R, Younger M. Lesser digit implants. Clin Podiatr Med Surg 2019;36(4): 651–61.
36. Alvine FG, Garvin KL. Peg and dowel fusion of the proximal interphalangeal joint. Foot Ankle 1980;1(2):90–4.
37. Magnan B, Bonetti I, Negri S, et al. Percutaneous distal osteotomy of lesser metatarsals (DMMO) for treatment of metatarsalgia with metatarsophalangeal instability. Foot Ankle Surg 2018;24(5):400–5.
38. Redfern D. Treatment of metatarsalgia with distal osteotomies. Foot Ankle Clin 2018;23(1):21–33.
39. Palma L de, Colonna E, Travasi M. The modified Jones procedure for pes cavovarus with claw hallux. J Foot Ankle Surg 1997;36(4):279–83.

Ankle Instability and Peroneal Disorders in Cavovarus Feet
Do I Need a Calcaneal Osteotomy?

Manfred Thomas, MD[a],*, Elena Delmastro, MD[b]

KEYWORDS

- Peroneal tendons • Cavovarus foot deformity • Ankle instability
- Calcaneus osteotomy • Tendon rupture

KEY POINTS

- Highest incidence for peroneal tendon lesion of all extra-articular lesions concomitant to lateral ligament lesion after ankle sprain.
- Cavovarus foot deformity as anatomic risk factor for chronic lateral ligament instability.
- Patient compliance important factor for treatment outcome.
- No clear threshold at what degree of deformity we need to treat a concomitant calcaneus varus deformity in cases of underlying ankle instability.

ANKLE INSTABILITY: DEFINITION AND CLASSIFICATION

Ankle sprains are one of the most common musculoskeletal injuries and occur at all levels of activities, accounting for nearly 40% of all sports injuries. Approximately 27,000 ankle sprains occur daily in the United States.[1] The most commonly injured structures are the lateral ligaments—mostly the talofibular and the calcaneofibular ligament. They have a high incidence of associated injuries as peroneal tendon rupture or dislocation, anterolateral impingement lesions or even osteochondral talar lesions.[2] Predisposing factors to lateral ankle sprains include hindfoot varus malalignment (outward rolling of the ankle during gait), tarsal coalition (limits balancing on uneven ground), or peroneal muscle weakness—secondary to previous injury or because of neurologic deficit—(reduces hindfoot eversion as counteract to inversion forces).[3,4]

In most cases of ligament lesions, the conservative management is sufficient. Nevertheless, the incidence of a chronic ankle instability after an acute ankle sprain is reported to be between 5% and 70%. There are different surgical techniques

[a] Department of Foot and Ankle Surgery, Hessingpark- Clinic, 1786199 Augsburg, Germany;
[b] Università Vita-Salute San Raffaele, Via Olgettina 58, 20132 Milano, Italy
* Corresponding author. Hessingpark-clinic, 1786199 Augsburg.
E-mail addresses: manfred.thomas71@outlook.com (M.T.); delmastro.elena@gmail.com (E.D.)

Foot Ankle Clin N Am 28 (2023) 759–773
https://doi.org/10.1016/j.fcl.2023.07.001
1083-7515/23/© 2023 Elsevier Inc. All rights reserved.

described for the treatment of a ligamentous instability. Anatomic or non-anatomic procedures are both reported to have good to excellent results in 81% to 97% of the cases.[2,5–9]

Instability recurrence may happen in an early or late stage; early recurrences usually follow an acute injury while late recurrences are more difficult to be defined because they have a more subtle development and pathogenesis.[6,8,10,11]

Surgical failure may result from different reasons. The Broström procedure indication, for example, is limited for cases of generalized ligamentous laxity, in longstanding instability or also in high-demand patients.[5,11–14] A specific onset in late chronic instability occurs because of a varus hindfoot malalignment.[15,16] With a rigid supinated hindfoot, a laterally shifted subtalar axis increases the supination moment and causes excessive inversion. Ankle and hindfoot varus are present in 8% of patients with primary instability and in 28% of patients requiring surgical therapy for such an instability.[12]

The subject of ankle instability is multicausative and depends on the tissue quality, the underlying anatomy and various other reasons.

CLINICAL EVALUATION

There should be a discrimination between acute and chronic lesions. In all cases, a thorough history of the accident, the frequency of ankle sprains in a chronic instability, and the possibility of walking after the sprain are also important information.

Especially in acute injuries, there might be a false-negative result during the acute first examination because of pain limiting the examination. Therefore, it is recommended to repeat the examination 48 hours after the injury, using the rest, ice, compression, elevation principle during that time frame.[10] There are 3 major parts of the examination.

1. Tenderness: tenderness alone does not help to detect a ligamentous lesion
2. Ecchymosis and hematoma (tenderness and hematoma together have a sensitivity of 90% to detect ligamentous injury)
3. Anterior drawer test (has a sensitivity of 90%, if all 3 tests are considered together, they have a sensitivity of 100%).

In chronic cases, the assessment of the foot should also include axis deviations on different levels of the leg; checkup for planus or cavus deformities; shortening of the calf muscle; and discrimination between fixed, rigid deformity, or flexible deformity.

The 2 most important tests are the anterior drawer test and the inversion stress test (talar tilt test).

In an unstable ankle joint, there will be typically a suction sign over the lateral gutter during the anterior drawer test (**Fig. 1**).

Precaution needs to be taken in case the tests are normal because this fact does not exclude instability.

RADIOGRAPHIC EVALUATION AND OTHER IMAGING

Standard ap and lateral weight-bearing radiographs should be performed to assess the tibiotalar angle, the Meary's angle, the calcaneal pitch angle (CIA), the Hibbs angle, the first metatarsal declination angle, the tibiocalcaneal angle, and lateral TC angle.[17] Those images also help to identify osteoarthritis, osteochondral defects, or other post-traumatic changes. An additional oblique foot radiograph is helpful in a cavus foot deformity (**Fig. 2**).

The Saltzman's view helps to define the Center of Rotation and Angulation (CORA) of axis deviation.[12]

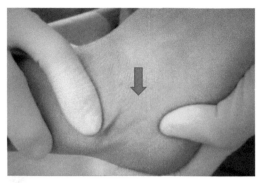

Fig. 1. Positive Drawer test with suction sign.

Ankle stress radiographs are controversial and are not commonly recommended, whereas the Broden's view in suspicion of a syndesmotic lesion or an abnormality of the posterior facet is helpful.

Full-length standing radiographs are used in suspicion of a more proximal deformity or axis deviation.

MRI is useful in suspicion of additional tendon or cartilage lesions and also if there is tenderness, swelling, and unclear suspicion of bony avulsion or ligament lesions (**Fig. 3**). Nowadays, a 3.0 T should be the MRI of choice. The disadvantage of MRI is that there are only very limited number of centers that can perform a dynamic MRI; otherwise, it is a static examination.

A weight-bearing computed tomography (CT) might be helpful in case of additional deformities, previous surgeries of the ankle or foot and or any additional abnormalities of the skeleton of the foot and ankle.[18,19]

Ultrasound could be useful in the hand of the experienced examiner for a dynamic examination of ligament and tendon injuries.[8,20,21]

Peroneal Tendon Disorders

Lesions and other pathologic conditions of the peroneal tendons are often underestimated or misdiagnosed. They are not rare after acute or even recurrent supination trauma of the ankle and may lead to persistent posterolateral ankle pain and/or severe functional limitations.[21,22]

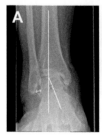 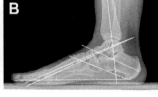 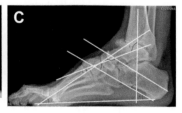

Fig. 2. (*A*): Weight-bearing Ankle AP with a varus tilt talus. X: tibiotalar angle; Y: lateral clear space. (*B*): Lateral view of a normal foot. (*C*): Lateral view of a cavus foot. Angle A: CIA. Angle B: Meary's angle. Angle C: Hibbs angle. Angle D: first metatarsal declination angle. Angle E: tibiotalar angle. Angle F: tibiocalcaneal angle. Angle G: lateral TC angle.

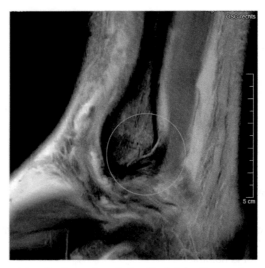

Fig. 3. MRI: bony avulsion fracture of posterior fibulotalar ligament.

There are 3 different categories of tendon lesions.

1. Tendinopathy including tendinitis/tenosynovitis/tendinosis
2. Subluxation or luxation/dislocation (**Fig. 4**).
3. Tendon tears and ruptures from partial to complete (**Fig. 5**).

In the active sports-population pathologies of the peroneal tendons are causing chronic lateral ankle pain, in up to 77% of the cases accompanied by chronic lateral instability. In case those patients need surgical repair, the overall finding is that in 33%

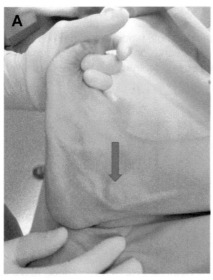
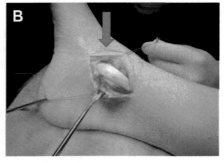

Fig. 4. (A): Peroneal tendon dislocation: (B): Peroneal tendon dislocation (intraoperative finding).

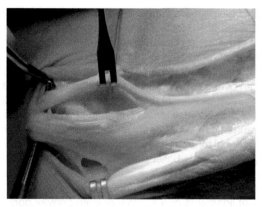

Fig. 5. Peroneal tendon longitudinal rupture.

of the group they also do need a lateral ligament repair. About 20% of the operated peroneal tendons show subluxation of the tendons, 10% show an abnormal flat dorsal groove of the fibula, and 33% show a far distally located muscle belly of the peroneus brevis muscle.[1,15,22]

Recurrent ankle supination trauma or chronic overuse may lead to hypertrophic tendinopathy, recurrent impingement, or interstitial tearing of the tendons. Tendinopathy is most often found in the areas of greatest stress and angular change—around the lateral malleolus (peroneus brevis), along the peroneal tubercle (**Fig. 6**) (peroneus brevis and longus) or within the cuboid groove (peroneus longus).

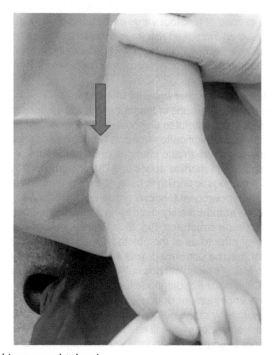

Fig. 6. Hypertrophic peroneal tubercle.

Isolated ruptures of the peroneal tendons are rare and are found mostly after severe supination trauma of the ankle joint. The relation between ruptures of the peroneus longus to peroneus brevis is 13% compared with 88%.[21,22] Lesions of both peroneal tendons are described in up to 38% of the patients.

The hindfoot alignment seems to be an important factor because cavovarus deformities may lead to an overload of the peroneal tendons, especially from the peroneus longus tendon[2,20,22] in up to 80% of the peroneal tendon pathologic conditions.

An impingement of the peroneal tendons is seen in cases of increased planovalgus deformity or posttraumatic heel deformity after calcaneus fractures.

Luxation of the peroneal tendons is relatively rare and occurs mainly after chronic or acute sports injury, for example ballet dancers or skiers. Chronic luxations are often associated with a chronic lateral ankle instability. Acute luxation is overseen or misdiagnosed as ligamentous injury in up to 40% of the cases.

Congenital laxity of ligaments or a shallow or even convex dorsal peroneal groove may lead to persistent tendon luxation. Because of recurrent tendon luxation, longitudinal tears of the tendons may occur.

Clinical presentation and assessment

Chronic peroneal tendon pathologic condition presents with dorsolateral pain, swelling, and tenderness over the peroneal groove. Muscle stress testing of the peroneals should always be performed bilaterally. In case of a split tendon or longitudinal tear of the tendon, a weakness is not commonly found unless the tear is chronic. Complete ruptures will lead to a loss of strength in the peroneal complex. Complete tears are much less common than the typical longitudinal tears, and a complete tear of both tendons is a rarity but it might happen. Peroneus brevis pathologic conditions mostly show complaints around the fibular tip or the retro malleolar groove, whereas peroneus longus pathologic conditions show mostly pain around the os peroneum and the cuboid groove. In case of hindfoot varus or metatarsus adductus or fixed plantarflexed first ray, there is an increased risk for medial shift of the hindfoot axis and secondary overload of the peroneal tendons and lateral ligaments. In all cases, the presence of a neurologic disorder or neuromuscular disease[15,22] should be excluded.

Radiographic evaluation and other imaging diagnostics

Routine weight-bearing radiographs of the foot and ankle ap and lateral and additional oblique views of the foot are helpful to diagnose any concomitant pathologic condition as pes cavus, fractures or calcifications of soft tissue, osteoarthritis changes, malalignment, congenital or posttraumatic changes of os peroneum or peroneal tubercle. On the ap radiograph or the mortise ap view, a "fleck sign" or "fibula sleeve avulsion fracture" (**Fig. 7**) is a diagnostic finding in case of a bony avulsion of the peroneal tendons or a luxation of the peroneal tendons grade III.[21]

MRI has become the standard diagnostic tool to evaluate the peroneal tendons and the surrounding soft tissue structures (**Fig. 8**) and has the advantage to also show the cartilage and ligament structures of the tibiotalar and the subtalar joint. In a few centers, a dynamic MRI may be performed, and it allows a more accurate diagnosis. To get advantage from today's technical possibilities, the use of a 3 T device is favorable.

Weight-bearing CT is helpful to diagnose the axis of the ankle and subtalar joint and also a possible bony impingement during weight-bearing.

Dynamic ultrasonography of the peroneal tendons helps to identify a subluxation or luxation of the peroneal tendons as well as chronic tears of the peroneal tendons. An experienced examiner taking the US and the use of a high-resolution ultrasonography is important for reproducible results.

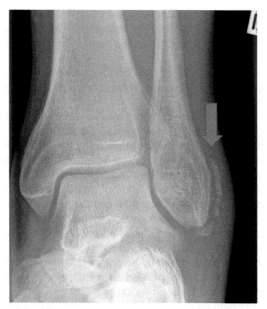

Fig. 7. Avulsion fracture after peroneal tendon luxation.

Cavus and Cavovarus Deformity Definition and Staging

In general, the cavus shape of the foot seems to be more common than estimated; there are reports with this finding in up to 20% to 25% of the population. The cavus foot shape resulting deformities are the result of an imbalance between intrinsic and

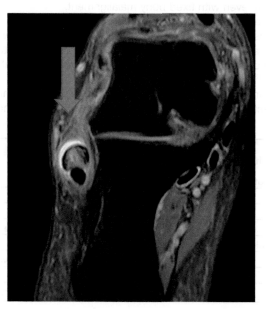

Fig. 8. MRI view of chronic tendinopathy of the peroneus brevis tendon.

extrinsic muscles. Cavovarus is a complex deformity,[13,14] which mostly occurs from muscle imbalance due to an underlying neurologic disorder (eg, Charcot-Marie-Tooth disease).[2,20,23,24] The possible causes leading to a cavovarus deformity are shown in **Table 1**.

Early onset of the disease during childhood aggravates the pathologic findings because of a disturbance of the growth of the bones with a disturbance of the entire forefoot and hindfoot anatomy.

For definition of the deformity, the relation between the hindfoot and the forefoot position during weight-bearing is crucial.[25] Fixed plantarflexion of the first ray may contribute to hindfoot varus (forefoot driven deformity), which will be aggravated if there is an additional weakness of the lateral ligaments. Medial and plantar medial peritalar subluxation with a strong overactive tibial posterior tendon and a weak peroneus brevis muscle results in a varus hindfoot malalignment and adduction of the midfoot and forefoot, which then is causing a medialized pulling vector of the Achilles tendon, which is also increasing the inversion moment and the varus deformity. In neurogenic cavovarus, there is a weak tibial anterior muscle, which becomes overpowered by the peroneus longus muscle, which is plantarflecting the first ray.[24] The amount of plantarflexion influences the height of the medial arch and determines the amount of cavus deformity. The plantarflexed first ray also influences the rotatory malalignment and causes the hyperpronation.

This rotatory component influences the position of the navicular, which shifts more dorsal than medial compared with the cuboid. With this movement, the Chopart joint becomes torqued and is fixing even more the hindfoot varus.

The plantar fascia, especially the medial bundle, is contracted and is adding the adduction and cavus component.

Several important discriminations and subspecifications of the cavovarus deformity are described. They need to get checked before deciding on a treatment strategy.[7,13,26]

Rigid or flexible deformity: Ranging from a subtle and flexible deformity (which may be tested clinically using the Coleman Block Test and dynamic functional tests)[19,27–29] to a rigid deformity even with fixed bony malalignment.

The clinical assessment proposed by Manoli and Graham and the use of determined radiological angles and views are very useful. Recently, the use of weight-bearing CT is considered as a helpful instrument for definition and for the setup of a treatment strategy (correlation of rotational midfoot deformity, hindfoot supination, and inframalleolar deformity).[18,30]

The development from a flexible to a rigid cavovarus foot is continuous and leads to a reduced contact area with the ground and concomitant to an increased localized

Table 1	
Causes of simple hindfoot varus malalignment	
Source of Hindfoot Varus	**Clinical Example**
-Knee	Medial osteoarthritis
-Lower leg	Malunited tibia fracture
-Supramalleolar	Malunited pilon fracture
-Tibiotalocalcaneal:	
Ankle joint	Chronic instability with varus osteoarthritis
Talocalcaneal	Tarsal coalition
Calcaneal	Malunited calcaneal fracture

Klammer et al., 2012.

pressure at the planta pedis with lateral overload and peak pressure below the heel and the metatarsals.

Because of the locking of the subtalar movement and the weakness of the peroneus brevis muscle, the capacity of shock absorption is impaired and the risk of lateral ankle instability is increased.[31] The fixed cavovarus deformity forces the talus into an increasing varus tilt with chronic varus overload and risk for the development of medial osteoarthritis.[12,16,20]

Clinical assessment

All lower leg axis and other deformities have to be defined in the patient standing barefoot and walking. The normal angle between the long axis of the leg and the axis of calcaneus is ranging from 0° neutral to 5° valgus. Any varus is pathologic. Callosities of the foot sole, the amount of plantarflexion of the first ray and the height of the medial arch must be checked. The position of the hindfoot, midfoot, and forefoot in valgus or varus stress must be observed. Moreover, the amount of rigidity of the deformity is an important parameter. The sign of a "peek-a-boo-heel"[16,30] (the medial aspect of the heel is seen when looking at the foot from frontal in standing position as shown in **Fig. 9**A), might be present and is only positive in a patient with varus heel position.[12,30]

The Coleman block-test[19,28] in patients with a plantarflexed first ray determines whether there is a forefoot-driven or a hindfoot-driven varus (the latter would be corrected with the Coleman block test, as shown in **Fig. 9**B). The Silfverskjöld test[25,29] is also an important tool to determine whether the gastroc-soleus complex is shortened. Another important examination is the testing of muscle strength of the peroneals, the

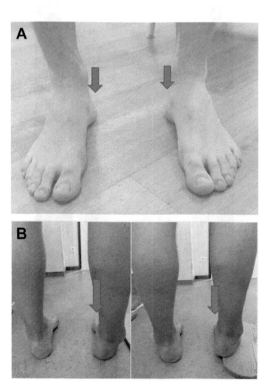

Fig. 9. (A): Peek-a-boo sign. (B): Coleman block test (picture by courtesy of Kris Buedts).

anterior tibial muscle and the gastroc-soleus muscles. Finally, the stability of the ankle and the subtalar joint and the lateral and the medial ligaments must be tested. Neurologic examination for muscle strength, sensation, and reflexes is completing the clinical assessment.

Radiographic assessment
As for the diagnosis of ankle instability, the standard radiographs should consist of a weight-bearing ap and lateral view of both ankles and feet and an additional oblique view of both feet. In addition, a Mortise view of the ankle should be obtained if ligamentous instability is suspected and a Broden's view if a subtalar instability is expected. Typically, there is a greater overlap of fibula and tibia in the Mortise view because the fibula is positioned more posterior due to the supramalleolar torsion and the hindfoot varus in the cavus foot.[17] The Saltzman view (**Fig. 10**) shows the correlation between the longitudinal axis of the tibia and the distance from that line crossing the cortex of the calcaneus to the lowest point of the calcaneus. This distance is on average 3.2 mm toward a heel valgus.[32]

The CT scan may be helpful in bony abnormalities as tarsal coalition or status post fracture, for example, fracture of the base of metatarsal IV or V.

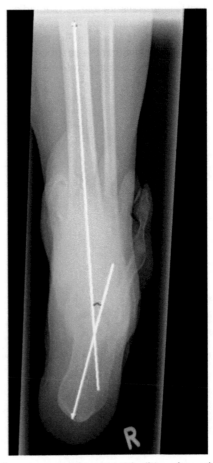

Fig. 10. Saltzman view in cavovarus deformity with tibio-calcaneal angle.

Nowadays, the weight-bearing CT has mostly overtaken the role of the CT scan, gives reproducible additional information for the preop planning, and helps to understand those deformities.[14,18,19]

The use of MRI is mainly helpful for the diagnosis of additional ligamentous injuries, cartilage injuries, or lesions of the peroneal tendons.

Clinical case

A 26-year-old male patient with cavovarus foot deformity, peroneus brevis tendinopathy, and acute rupture of fibulocalcanear ligament (**Fig. 11**).

The patient showed the same deformity on the other foot (pain free) and refused therefore surgical treatment on the injured side.

The Role of Calcaneal Osteotomies in Inframalleolar Cavovarus Deformities

The calcaneus osteotomy as treatment in a cavus or cavovarus foot deformity has to be seen as part of a complex treatment strategy.[20,33] Depending on the additionally presented soft tissue problems, the treatment consists of several surgical steps.[2,34] If the CORA is below the ankle joint, a calcaneus osteotomy needs to be considered. Numerous techniques are described.[20,25,33,35]

The most popular technique is the Dwyer osteotomy: a lateral oblique closing wedge osteotomy of the calcaneus with a subsequent lateralization of the tuberosity. The disadvantages of this procedure are a calcaneus shortening and (in cases of severe deformities with a large wedge resection) a weakness of the triceps because of the change of the Achilles tendon lever arm.

The lateralizing osteotomy is the most used type of osteotomy and allows a high amount of shifting. The disadvantage is the possible impairment of the tarsal tunnel with a resulting nerve compression and the limited possibility of rotational corrections.

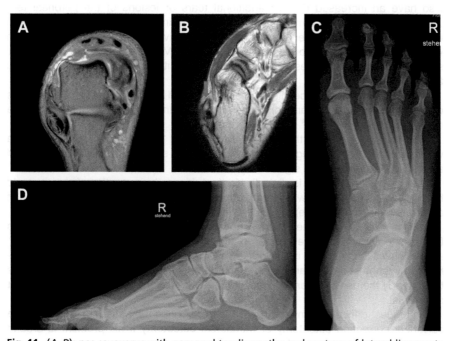

Fig. 11. (*A–D*): pes cavovarus with peroneal tendinopathy and rupture of lateral ligaments.

The Z-shaped osteotomy allows the highest amount of correction in 3 dimensions. It allows a rotational component and several corrections with additional possibility to lengthen or shorten the calcaneus.

Although correcting a hindfoot varus with an inframalleolar pathologic condition, the calcaneus osteotomy is an important part of the surgical treatment.

More difficult is the role of osteotomies in the combination of inframalleolar and supramalleolar deformity. In that case, the surgical approach is more extensive. In those cases, the calcaneus correction is depending on the amount of the deformity and is an important part of the correction of pathology. It also helps to ensure the success of additional correction of ankle instability and peroneal tendon disorders (if combined with the hindfoot cavus).[2,20,36]

SUMMARY

Several studies show that ankle instability presents often with additional findings as hindfoot varus, peroneal tendon lesions, os trigonum syndrome, lateral gutter ossicles, anterior tibial spurs, or tarsal coalition.[4,16] Peroneal tendon lesions are often not recognized but are still described with an incidence of 25% in patients with a lateral ligament instability. They are mostly missed at the time of the first presentation in the outpatient clinic.[3,21,22]

However, in patients presenting with a diagnosed peroneal tendon pathologic condition, about 75% of the cases present with an additional chronic lateral ankle instability.[15,21,22]

Whereas there is a subtle cavus deformity of the heel described in about 10% of the population and the patients with a lateral ankle instability do show a significant percentage of inframalleolar hindfoot varus, there are clear signs for an increased risk for lateral ankle instability in patients with a varus heel.[1,27,30] Those patients also have an increased risk for additional tears or lesions of the peroneal tendons.[21,22] The clinical examination helps to determine on which level is the lateral instability and also whether there is a hindfoot-driven varus or a forefoot-driven varus and whether the deformity is flexible or rigid. MRI in combination with clinical symptoms shows the highest sensitivity and specificity for the diagnosis of peroneal tendon tears.

In the last years, weight-bearing CT has become an important tool for the diagnosis of the degree of deformity and for further understanding of the different elements of a cavovarus deformity.[14,18,24]

If the heel does not show the physiologic position of 1° to 5° of valgus but presents a varus position of various degrees, the risk of an ankle sprain with the additional risk of a peroneal tendon lesion is significantly increased.

If the cavus or cavovarus is clinically hindfoot driven, the correction of choice would be a calcaneus osteotomy with lateralization of the distal fragment and/or resection of a lateral wedge (Dwyer type).[2,20]

There is no clear recommendation of how much to shift or of how thick the wedge in Dwyer osteotomy should be in order to achieve a perfect correction.

If the cavus or cavovarus is forefoot driven, the plantarflexed first ray has to be corrected by lengthening or transferring of the peroneus longus tendon to the peroneus brevis or by the use of a dorsal extending osteotomy in the proximal third of the first metatarsal.[2,4,12]

The biggest difficulty in my experience is to convince the patient of the need for a calcaneal correction osteotomy or metatarsal osteotomy if his problem is around the ankle and not around the heel.

The most common situation in our patients is the case of bilateral symmetric hind-foot varus with only one side having a problem and the other ankle and hindfoot presenting without symptoms but with the same deformity. This situation is usually giving the surgeon a hard time to explain the patient why he needs to undergo a surgical intervention.

We definitely need clinical and biomechanical studies to proof how much the corrected hindfoot axis is supporting an unstable ankle with peroneal lesions. We need to find a tool for definition of the necessary degree of hindfoot and forefoot correction to reduce an underlying hindfoot malalignment and to help prevent further ligamentous and tendinous lesions in the further natural course of the pathology.

Clinical and biomechanical studies are important for further understanding of the needed amount of correction for the different pathologic conditions. The use of weight-bearing CT will help us to better understand the effects of correction of the deformity at different levels in the hindfoot and forefoot.

CLINICS CARE POINTS

- In approximately 25% of the patients with chronic lateral ankle instability, there is high incidence of additional peroneal tendon pathologic condition, more frequent with tears of the peroneus brevis than tears of peroneus longus tendon.

- Discrimination between rigid and flexible hindfoot varus deformity and definition of the level of deformity is crucial for further treatments.

- Discrimination between hindfoot-driven and forefoot-driven cavus foot is essential for further treatment strategies.

- Patients with cavus foot deformities are more likely to get an ankle instability than a peroneal tendon disorder.

DISCLOSURE

The authors have nothing to disclose.

REFERENCES

1. Franson J, Baravarian B. Lateral ankle triad: the triple injury of ankle synovitis, lateral ankle instability, and peroneal tendon tear. Clin Podiatr Med Surg 2011; 28(1):105–15.
2. Bariteau JT, Blankenhorn BD, Tofte JN, et al. What is the role and limit of calcaneal osteotomy in the cavovarus foot? Foot Ankle Clin 2013;18(4):697–714.
3. Larsen E, Angermann P. Association of ankle instability and foot deformity. Acta Orthop Scand 1990;61(2):136–9.
4. Strauss JE, Forsberg JA, Lippert FG 3rd. Chronic lateral ankle instability and associated conditions: a rationale for treatment. Foot Ankle Int 2007;28(10): 1041–4.
5. Colville MR. Surgical treatment of the unstable ankle. J Am Acad Orthop Surg 1998;6(6):368–77.
6. Gibboney MD, Dreyer MA. Lateral Ankle Instability. In: StatPearls. Treasure Island (FL): StatPearls Publishing; 2023.
7. Hansen JRT. Cavus foot. Saxena A. International Advances in foot and ankle Surgery. London: Springer; 2011.

8. Ruiz R, Hintermann B. Foot and ankle instability: a clinical guide to diagnosis and surgical management. Springer; 2021.

9. Tourné Y, Mabit C. Lateral ligament reconstruction procedures for the ankle. Orthop Traumatol Surg Res 2017;103(1S):S171–81.

10. Chan KM, Karlsson J, Van Dijk CN. Diagnosis of the ankle sprain: history and physical examination; Paper presented at the international society of Arthroscopy, Knee Surgery and Orthopaedic Sports Medicine- International Federation of Sports Medicine (ISAKOS- FIMS). World Consensus Conference on Ankle Instability January 2005;21.

11. Freeman MA. Instability of the Foot after injuries to the lateral ligaments of the ankle. J Bone Joint Surg Br 1965;47(4):669–77.

12. Fortin PT, Guettler J, Manoli A 2nd. Idiopathic cavovarus and lateral ankle instability: recognition and treatment implications relating to ankle arthritis. Foot Ankle Int 2002;23(11):1031–7.

13. Krähenbühl N, Weinberg MW. Anatomy and Biomechanics of Cavovarus Deformity. Foot Ankle Clin 2019;24(2):173–81.

14. Ranjit S, Sangoi D, Cullen N, et al. Assessing the coronal plane deformity in Charcot Marie Tooth Cavovarus feet using automated 3D measurements. Foot Ankle Surg 2023. https://doi.org/10.1016/j.fas.2023.02.013. S1268-7731(23)00044-9.

15. Redfern D, Myerson M. The management of concomitant tears of the peroneus longus and brevis tendons. Foot Ankle Int 2004;25(10):695–707.

16. Shim DW, Suh JW, Park KH, et al. Diagnosis and Operation Results for Chronic lateral Ankle Instability with subtle Cavovarus Deformity and a Peek-A-Boo Heel Sign. Yonsei Med J 2020;61(7):635–9.

17. Osher L, Shook JE. Imaging of the Pes Cavus Deformity. Clin Podiatr Med Surg 2021;38(3):303–21.

18. Bernasconi A, Cooper L, Lyle S, et al. Intraobserver and interobserver reliability of cone beam weightbearing semi-automatic three-dimensional measurements in symptomatic pes cavovarus. Foot Ankle Surg 2020;26(5):564–72.

19. Foran IM, Mehraban N, Jacobsen SK, et al. Impact of Coleman Block Test on Adult Hindfoot Alignment Assessed by Clinical Examination, Radiography, and Weight-Bearing Computed Tomography. Foot Ankle Orthop 2020;5(3). 2473011 420933264.

20. Usuelli FG, Manzi L. Inframalleolar Varus Deformity: Role of Calcaneal Osteotomies. Foot Ankle Clin 2019;24(2):219–37.

21. Willegger M, Hirtler L, Schwarz GM, et al. Peronealsehnenpathologien : Von der Diagnose bis zur Behandlung [Peroneal tendon pathologies : From the diagnosis to treatment]. Orthopä 2021;50(7):589–604. German.

22. van Dijk PAD, Kerkhoffs GMMJ, Chiodo C, et al. Chronic Disorders of the Peroneal Tendons: Current Concepts Review of the Literature. J Am Acad Orthop Surg 2019;27(16):590–8.

23. López-López D, Larrainzar-Garijo R, Becerro-de-Bengoa-Vallejo R, et al. Effectiveness of calcaneal osteotomy in surgical treatment of foot conditions: A Prisma statement guidelines compliant systematic review. Int Wound J 2022;19(6):1494–501.

24. Waldman LE, Michalski MP, Giaconi JC, et al. Charcot-Marie-Tooth Disease of the Foot and Ankle: Imaging Features and Pathophysiology. Radiographics 2023;43(4). e220114.

25. Klammer G, Benninger E, Espinosa N. The varus ankle and instability. Foot Ankle Clin 2012;17(1):57–82.

26. DiDomenico LA, Abdelfattah S, Chan D, et al. The Cavovarus Ankle: Approaches to Ankle Instability and Inframalleolar Deformity. Clin Podiatr Med Surg 2021; 38(3):461–81.
27. Chilvers M, Manoli A 2nd. The subtle cavus foot and association with ankle instability and lateral foot overload. Foot Ankle Clin 2008;13(2):315–24, vii.
28. Coleman SS, Chesnut WJ. A simple test for hindfoot flexibility in the cavovarus foot. Clin Orthop Relat Res 1977;(123):60–2.
29. Krause F, Seidel A. Malalignment and Lateral Ankle Instability: Causes of Failure from the Va Tibia to the Cavovarus Foot. Foot Ankle Clin 2018;23(4):593–603.
30. Manoli A 2nd, Graham B. The subtle cavus foot, "the underpronator". Foot Ankle Int 2005;26(3):256–63.
31. Vienne P, Schöniger R, Helmy N, et al. Hindfoot instability in cavovarus deformity: static and dynamic balancing. Foot Ankle Int 2007;28(1):96–102.
32. Saltzman CL, el-Khoury GY. The hindfoot alignment view. Foot Ankle Int 1995; 16(9):572–6.
33. Wolfe JR, McKee TD, Nicholes M. Use of Calcaneal Osteotomies in the Correction of Inframalleolar Cavovarus Deformity. Clin Podiatr Med Surg 2021;38(3):379–89.
34. Kaplan JRM, Aiyer A, Cerrato RA, et al. Operative Treatment of the Cavovarus Foot. Foot Ankle Int 2018;39(11):1370–82.
35. Hintermann B, Knupp M, Barg A. Joint-preserving surgery of asymmetric ankle osteoarthritis with peritalar instability. Foot Ankle Clin 2013;18(3):503–16.
36. Usuelli FG, Mason L, Grassi M, et al. Lateral ankle and hindfoot instability: a new clinical based classification. Foot Ankle Surg 2014;20(4):231–6.

Posterior Heel Pain in Cavovarus Foot

How to Approach It

Conor Moran, MD, Yves Tourné, MD, PhD*

KEYWORDS

- Cavovarus • Heel pain • Achilles tendinopathy • Haglund's syndrome
- Calcaneal osteotomy

KEY POINTS

- Heel pain in cavovarus foot is a constellation of pathologies that can present in the same way but must be addressed individually and appropriately.
- Haglund's syndrome and variants involve multiple aspects; the position and morphology of the calcaneus can impinge on the surrounding soft tissues, causing overtension in the calf and Achilles tendinopathy, as well as retrocalcaneal bursitis and even pressure under the forefoot.
- Addressing the various aspects of the syndrome can be done in a multitude of ways but must be tailored to the patient's individual needs.
- A lateral weightbearing x-ray of the ankle combined with an MRI of the distal end of the Achilles tendon are key aspects of the workup for decision-making and diagnosis.
- More often than not, surgical treatment is required to achieve a positive outcome.

INTRODUCTION

The cavus foot describes a spectrum of feet characterized by a high medial arch. This high arch can be driven by a number of different factors, including a high calcaneal pitch, a plantarflexed forefoot, or an excessive bend in the midfoot. Cavus feet affect roughly one-quarter of the population.[1] There can be a varus position of the hindfoot associated with the increased calcaneal pitch.[2,3] There are a number of associated pathologies with cavovarus foot, such as Charcot Marie Tooth, Little disease, and other neurological disorders; however, these are beyond the scope of this article, which will focus on primary morphological cavus foot.

The position of the calcaneus in the cavovarus foot can have several pathological implications for the posterior heel. Previously described "Haglund's syndrome and

Centre Osteo Articulaires des Cèdres, 5 Rue des Tropiques Echirolles 38130, France
* Corresponding author.
E-mail address: ytme@me.com

Foot Ankle Clin N Am 28 (2023) 775–789
https://doi.org/10.1016/j.fcl.2023.06.001
1083-7515/23/© 2023 Elsevier Inc. All rights reserved.

variants"[4,5] demonstrate an impingement process between the posterior tuberosity of the calcaneus and the surrounding soft tissues. Haglund's deformity itself is characterized by a posterosuperior bony prominence of the calcaneus.[6,7] The tendon inserts distal to the posterior tuberosity of the calcaneus, as well as on the medial and lateral aspects. Between the distal Achilles tendon and the posterior tuberosity, immediately proximal to the insertion is the retrocalcaneal bursa,[8] a distinct anatomical entity interposed between the anterior surface of the Achilles tendon and the posterior surface of the calcaneal tuberosity in the posteroinferior corner of the retrocalcaneal recess.[9] This anatomy leaves both the bursa[7] and the tendon liable to impingement between the tendon and the bony prominence,[10] especially in the cavus position with a high calcaneal pitch, with or without a Haglund's deformity, where the Achilles tendon is tented over the posterior tuberosity to insert on what becomes the inferior surface. It is commonly seen that individuals with a cavovarus foot have a positive Silfverskiöld's test due to overtension of the calf muscles.

Overtension of the posterior kinetic chain and the gastrosoleus complex coupled with impingement can cause pain. The most common causes are insertional Achilles tendinopathy, Haglund's disease or enthesopathy, or retrocalcaneal bursitis.[11] Prevalence ranges from 6.5% to 18% in runners and 9% in dancers.[12] Risk factors for injury to the Achilles tendon are decreased blood supply with advancing age, corticosteroid or fluroquinolone use, and male sex; external risk factors include high-intensity plyometric exercises, training on unfamiliar surfaces, or incorrect footwear.[13]

WORKUP

The workup of "Haglund's syndromes" and variants involves a full history and clinical examination. Etiologic studies have suggested an increased incidence of insertional Achilles tendinopathy with systemic issues such as hypertension, diabetes, obesity, and hormone replacement therapy.[14] Lifestyle factors such as increased activity such as walking or running and increased pressure caused by a shoe heel counter can play an aggravating role, and the use of fluroquinolones has been related to Achilles tendinopathy and rupture.[15]

On physical examination, a prominence can be felt medial and lateral to the Achilles tendon insertion, and tenderness can be located centrally or globally on the posterior heel.[11] Symptoms associated with retrocalcaneal bursitis, such as local inflammation and swelling, may occur concurrently.

Weightbearing x-rays allow analysis of the bony configuration and Meary's angle. Meary's angle is subtended between a line drawn along the longitudinal axes of the talus and the first metatarsal on a standard lateral weightbearing x-ray. An angle of > 4 degrees convex upwards indicates a cavus deformity. This line also allows for the determination of where in the foot the deformity occurs. The lateral weightbearing x-ray may also reveal insertional proliferative spurring (**Fig. 1**) and intratendinous calcifications, as well as the presence of a Haglund's deformity (**Fig. 2**). The radiographic findings allow assessment of the bony measurements.[16,17] Previously, the X/Y ratio has been described that measures if a calcaneus is long superiorly[4] (**Fig. 3**). The superiorly long calcaneus predisposes to insertional tendon difficulties as the tendon is tented more dramatically over the posterior tuberosity to reach its insertion inferiorly, thus has a longer course and puts increased tension through the posterior kinetic chain. A ratio under 2.5 is considered abnormal.

Other radiographic measurements have been described[18–20]; however, these show poor specificity and reliability, excepted the pitch angle of Ruch. A pitch angle of Ruch is considered abnormal when over 20°.

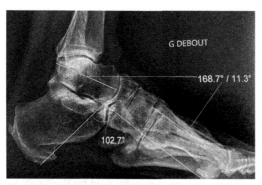

Fig. 1. Lateral weightbearing radiograph of the foot showing a Meary's angle of 11.3 indicating cavus, with prominent calcaneal spurs at the insertion of the Achilles tendon and the plantar fascia attachment.

Anteroposterior view using the Meary view (**Fig. 4**), the Salzman view, and the long axial view is helpful to assess the hindfoot alignment, and even the use of weightbearing computed tomography tends to provide a more accurate evaluation of the deformity.[21–24]

Ultrasound is a nonexpensive, noninvasive imaging modality that can be rapidly performed, often in-office in experienced hands, that can reveal tendon thickening as well as retrocalcaneal bursitis.[25]

MRI should be routinely performed to assess the soft tissues. The MRI scan allows assessment of the tendon itself; it will show focal microtears (**Fig. 5**). It also allows confirmation of the clinical examination findings of insertional versus corporeal tendonitis. The tendon insertion site can be assessed based on the percentage of tendon involved and the quality of the remaining tendon, on horizontal slices.[26]

DIFFERENTIAL DIAGNOSIS/SO-CALLED POSTERIOR HEEL PAIN

The differential diagnosis of posterior heel pain beyond the Achilles tendon should not be forgotten. Cavovarus feet can also lead to lateral ankle instability through recurrent sprains and rupture of the lateral ligamentous complex.[27,28] This can then lead to peroneal tendonitis and cartilage damage at the level of the ankle, which can also be sources of posterior heel pain. A tight posterior kinetic chain common in cavovarus

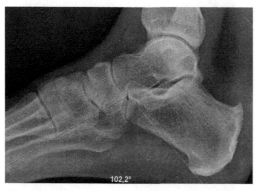

Fig. 2. Lateral weightbearing view of the posterior foot showing a prominence at the posterosuperior aspect of the calcaneus—Haglund's deformity.

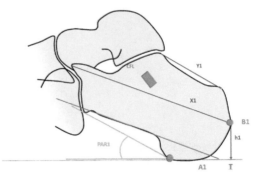

Fig. 3. Radiographic reproducible measurements used for Haglund's syndrome to assess the calcaneus shape. The X/Y ratio is normally over 2.5 and the pitch angle of Ruch (PAR) is under 20°.

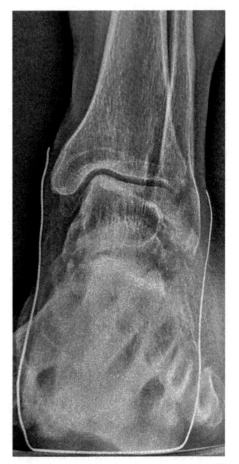

Fig. 4. Frontal view using the Meary evaluation to assess the hindfoot varus alignment.

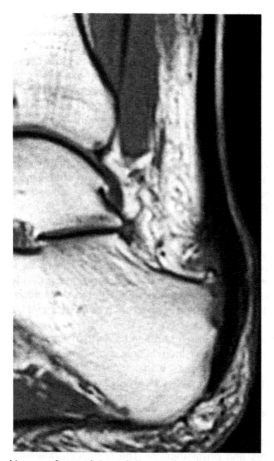

Fig. 5. T1-weighted image of MRI of the Achilles tendon showing the microtears (bright) in the body of the tendon at the insertion site and local inflammation resulting from impingement between the bone and tendon.

feet can also result in plantar fasciitis, which can co-exist with Achilles pathology due to tension on both sides of the calcaneal posterior lever arm. Other pathologies that can present with posterior heel pain include noninsertional Achilles tendinopathy, flexor hallucis longus (FHL) tendinopathy, os trigonum/talus posterior process stress fracture, and calcaneus stress fracture. Posterior tibial tendon tendinopathy or insufficiency causing adult-acquired flat foot with impingement or arthritis in the ankle or posterior facet of the subtalar joint can also present as posterior heel pain, but these are beyond the scope of this article and are addressed elsewhere.

CONSERVATIVE MANAGEMENT

Management of posterior heel pain and Achilles tendonitis is guided by the position and severity of the condition. Corporeal or noninsertional tendinopathy is rarely a surgical condition and is effectively treated with rest, ice, compression, and physiotherapy concentric and eccentric exercises as per the Stanish protocol.

Other conservative management options include lifestyle changes such as weight loss and activity modification. Further interventions will be introduced such as orthotics, such as a heel raise to decrease stretch on the Achilles tendon or a more bespoke Achilles support device,[29] open-backed shoes to avoid compression, cryotherapy, topical analgesics, or systemic anti-inflammatories[11]

Corticosteroid injections in or around the Achilles tendon must be undertaken with caution in insertional Achilles tendinopathy as they have been shown to increase the risk of ruptures,[30,31] and systematic reviews have shown significant long-term harms to tendon tissue and cells associated with glucocorticoid injections,[32] as well as an increased risk of wound infection in any subsequent operative intervention. There are persisting studies with some mild evidence that noninsertional tendinopathy can have improved outcomes by combining ultrasound-guided corticosteroid injection with exercise therapy,[33] especially in those with inflammatory arthropathies.[34]

Platelet-rich plasma (PRP) injection is another form of conservative treatment that has been tried; however, a recent systematic review showed no significant benefit with the use of PRP injections[35]

Retrocalcaneal bursitis is often associated with other pathologies of the posterior heel. Patients will describe pain in the back of the heel, often anterior to the Achilles tendon, especially on plantarflexion of the foot. Van Sterkenburg and colleagues[36] found a high degree of interobserver and intraobserver reliability for the diagnosis of retrocalcaneal bursitis due to the loss of the sharp edges of Kager's triangle on the lateral weightbearing x-rays of the ankle. Although this is insufficient to rule out other co-existing pathologies, soft tissue imaging such as MRI is more beneficial to view the tendon.

There is some evidence for image-guided steroid injection in the case of isolated retrocalcaneal bursitis; however, there is only short-term follow-up.[37] Boone and colleagues reported excellent results with image-guided injection for retrocalcaneal bursitis; however, they noted 4 incidences of acute tendon rupture out of 218 cases,[38–40] and again caution would be advised because of the high rate of tendon rupture.

Although noninsertional tendinopathy is wholly treated by nonoperative means, there can also be a role for conservative management of insertional tendonitis. This can be treated initially by a short period of immobilization followed by gradual introduction of activities and physiotherapy. The condition, however, requires surgical intervention when it becomes chronic and debilitating.

OPERATIVE INTERVENTION/SURGICAL MANAGEMENT

There are a number of surgical interventions to alleviate the pain. The choice of surgery depends on the specific morphology and causative factors of the patient's pain. Osseus interventions should be considered first to correct any deformities that may cause the pain, as if left unaddressed, the pathology will recur, and then soft tissue anomalies can be addressed to repair or reconstruct the tendon.

1. Osseus interventions
   The calcaneus osteotomies are designed to decrease impingement on the Achilles tendon over Haglund's deformity and reduce its excursion.
   a. Calcaneoplasty is a remodeling of the posterior aspect of the calcaneus by osteotomy and removal of the posterosuperior aspect of the calcaneus, therefore reducing impingement on the tendon[41]
      Open—traditionally, calcaneoplasty is done open, either from a lateral incision or, if performed in conjunction with a tendonous procedure it can be done from the posterior aspect prior to tendon reattachment
      Percutaneous–A recent systematic review has demonstrated that endoscopic calcaneoplasty has less complications, a more rapid return to sporting

activities (11.9 ± 0.3 weeks vs 20.7 ± 3.3 weeks for open techniques), and a significantly better improvement in AOFAS scores than open techniques.[42]

b. The Zadek osteotomy is a dorsal closing wedge osteotomy of the calcaneus. Stabilization is performed by compressive screws or a lateral plate (**Fig. 6**). This osteotomy is designed to reduce the pressure of the posterosuperior aspect of the calcaneus on the tendon, while at the same time decreasing the tendon excursion length by rotating the insertion site of the tendon into a slightly more superior position. It can be appropriately performed when the X/Y ratio is less than 2.5 and the pitch angle is greater than 20°.[4,5,43–46] The effect of the Zadek osteotomy consists of reducing the lever arm on the tendon. This technique leads to improvement in ankle dorsiflexion and thus decreases the excessive tensile stress on the distal end of the Achilles tendon, which is correlated to excellent functional scores[43] (**Fig. 7**).

   The Zadek osteotomy is traditionally performed via an extended lateral incision allowing subperiosteal access to the lateral aspect of the calcaneus, extending up to the insertion of the Achilles tendon, this allows decompression of the retrocalcaneal bursa at the same time, and if there is a significantly exaggerated Haglund's deformity, simultaneous calcaneoplasty is performed.[5]

   MIS Percutaneous Zadek has also been described with the use of a 3 × 20 mm cutting burr and a 3 mm wedge burr through a small laterally based skin incision.[47–49] There are fewer wound complications relating to MIS; however, surgeon experience with the technique has a significant impact on outcomes.[50]

c. Additional deformities of the cavus foot can and should be addressed at this time. An accentuated varus position of the calcaneus causes the Achilles to be pulled away from the midline and gives a line of action further into varus (**Fig. 8**). The varus deformity can affect the stability of the hindfoot, increasing the stress forces on the lateral soft tissues, such as the collateral lateral ligament and the peroneal tendons as well[27,28] (**Fig. 9**).

   The varus aspect of the calcaneus can be addressed with a lateralizing osteotomy of the calcaneus such as a Dwyer or a Malerba osteotomy[51,52] (**Fig. 10**).

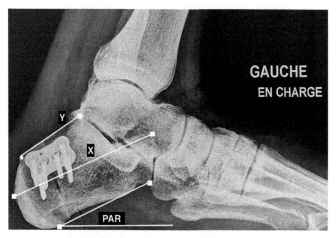

Fig. 6. Postoperative radiograph of a calcaneus post-Zadek procedure held with a 6-hole plate. The osteotomy line is clearly visible.

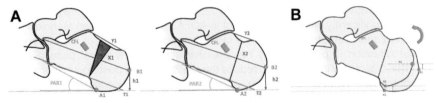

Fig. 7. (*A, B*) Biomechanical principles related to the surgical procedure: (*A*) Modifications of the calcaneus shape resulting of the Zadek's osteotomy (*grey triangle*). The X/Y ratio of Tourné moves from under 2.5 (X1/Y1) to over 2.5 (X2/Y2). The pitch angle of Ruch is higher preoperatively (PAR1) than postoperatively (PAR2). (*B*) Due to the osteotomy, point A moves dorsally from its A1 position to the A2 one. Similarly, the insertion point of the Achilles tendon on to the calcaneus, (*B*), moves from its position B1 to B2. Those modifications induce a reduction of the level arm of the Achilles tendon.

A Zadek osteotomy can be combined to a Dwyer one when performing a wedge in 2 planes, lateral and AP, although evidence of this being widely practiced in the literature is scarce.

If the varus calcaneus is forefoot driven, there can be metatarsalgia under the head of the first metatarsal due to increased pressure. This can be addressed with a dorsal closing wedge osteotomy of the first ray, if the clinical picture is indicative.

2. Procedures involving the soft tissues

Soft tissue procedures are utilized to repair or reconstruct tears or partial tears of the Achilles tendon and local inflammation.

a. Retrocalcaneal bursitis—excision of the inflamed bursa at the time of more extensive intervention can provide additional pain relief[53]

b. Spurs resection: disconnection/reattachment of the Achilles tendon

When the Achilles tendon is placed under long-term increased tension, it can undergo hypertrophic changes at the insertion site that result in spur formation (**Fig. 11**). When performing a debridement of the diseased portion of the Achilles tendon, these spurs are commonly debrided. Some authors prefer to

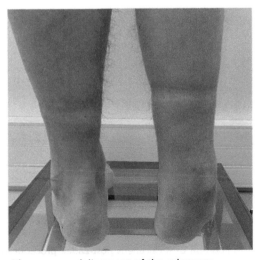

Fig. 8. Cavus foot with a varus malalignment of the calcaneus.

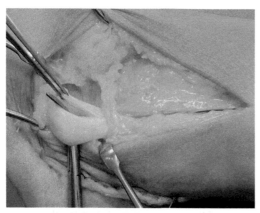

Fig. 9. Longitudinal chronic tear on the Peroneus brevis tendon.

leave a portion of the tendon in continuity with its insertion site in order to be able to repair it with appropriate length, and some detach completely.[53,54] There are multiple methods of reattaching the tendon to the bone, including the double-row speed-bridge system, which can be done by open[55–57](**Fig. 12**) or percutaneous technique.[58] Nevertheless, depending on the size and orientation of the spurs and the quality of the distal end of the Achilles tendon, in most cases, the spurs can be left alone; the decompression and the decrease of the lever arm on the insertional part of the Achilles tendon, induced by the Zadek osteotomy, is efficient on its own.

c. Augmentation of the distal-end Achilles tendon—If the distal end of the Achilles tendon has become too damaged and greater than 30% of the tendon has become detached from the bone, it is recommended to debride the tendon and augment the repair using a tendon transfer; this is commonly done using the FHL.[59,60] Plantaris is also readily used to augment the repair if available.

d. Achilles tendon elongation. In the cavovarus foot, the nature of the calcaneal pitch and the posteroinferior insertion of the tendon is such that the Achilles is under increased tension. Thus, affected individuals will commonly have reduced

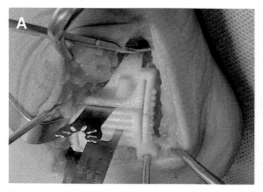
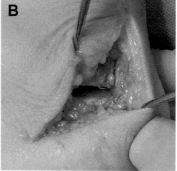

Fig. 10. (*A, B*) Intraoperative pictures during a Malerba osteotomy procedure. (*A*) Patient-specific instrumentation technology performed using 3-dimensional computed tomography scan reconstruction. (*B*) The Z shape of this closing wedge osteotomy before fixation.

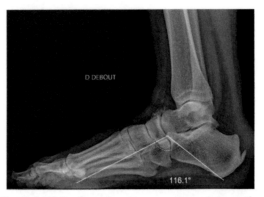

Fig. 11. Lateral radiograph of the foot showing an enthesophyte at the Achilles insertion, due to osseus hypertrophy of the ligament tissue increasing the impingement at the posterior aspect of the heel.

dorsiflexion of the ankle and may have increased pressure points under the forefoot. One approach to decrease the tension in the Achilles tendon is to increase the length. There are numerous ways of doing this each with their advantages and disadvantages.

The Achilles tendon can be lengthened directly, commonly via a 3-incision percutaneous technique or via a z-lengthening technique. This has the advantage of lengthening both the gastrocnemius and the soleus at the same time as they both insert via the Achilles tendon; however, this can be detrimental if preoperatively the dorsiflexion of the ankle is augmented by bending the knee and taking the gastrocnemius out of the equation. This must be assessed carefully via Silfverskiöld's test.

To lengthen the gastrocnemius in isolation, there are several methods at several different points in the calf. The two most common being the Strayer procedure, where the gastrocnemius fascia is released below the muscle belly, roughly at the junction of the proximal two-thirds and the distal one-third of the calf. This method has up to 38% complication rate, predominately nerve injury from the adjacent sural nerve.[61] The other common method of lengthening the gastrocnemius is to release the medial head at the posterior knee. This has the

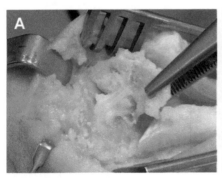
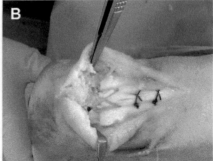

Fig. 12. (*A, B*) Disconnection/reattachment of the Achilles tendon. (*A*) The distal end of the Achilles tendon is divided in 2 bundles and completely detached. The spur is removed. (*B*) The tendon is reattached using a double-row speed-bridge system.

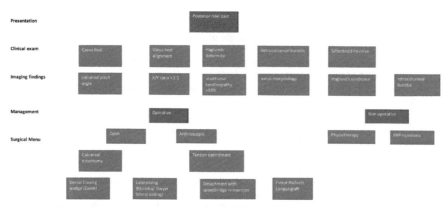

Fig. 13. Table outlining the broad treatment algorithm for someone who presents with posterior heel pain relating to Haglund's syndrome and variants.

advantage of not needing to put the patient in a cast afterward and can be done quickly and bilaterally simultaneously with immediate rehab.[62]

Patients who have undergone Zadek osteotomy also benefit from the "lengthening effect" provided by the rotation of the Achilles insertion point, and this could be enough to relax the gastrosoleus complex.[43]

SUMMARY

There are a constellation of pathologies involved in Haglund's syndrome and variants. Each of these must be addressed in order to appropriately treat the patient, allow them to return to their activities of daily living, and return to the level of sports they once enjoyed. As with any treatment plan, conservative management should be exhausted prior to embarking on operative intervention; however, there is a strong argument for surgery.

Both bony and soft tissue abnormalities must be addressed, and the surgical menu to address each should be selected accordingly. The overall morphology of the foot must be examined clinically and radiologically. The calcaneal pitch, the X/Y angle, the presence of Haglund's deformity, and the degree of varus will inform the surgeon if an osteotomy on the calcaneus or calcaneoplasty should be performed and to what degree. The MRI scan will inform the surgeon of the degree of involvement of the tendon itself, and therefore as to whether a tendon transfer or a speed-bridge repair should be performed.

Although there are a number of different methods of performing these procedures, minimally invasive versus endoscopic versus open, each technique has its advantages and disadvantages. The adage remains that the surgery that gets the best results for the patient is the operation with which the surgeon is most comfortable.

The most important factor when dealing with posterior heel pain in the cavovarus foot is that the time is taken to appropriately diagnose all the causative factors for the pathology and address each of them (**Fig. 13**).

CLINICS CARE POINTS

Pearls
- Several different pathologies can present with pain in the posterior heel, especially in the middle-aged athlete

- Evaluate the Achilles tendon carefully, as well as the position and morphology of the calcaneus. If there is an increased pitch angle or an X/Y ratio less than 2.5, the patient may benefit from an osteotomy to address this
- A Zadek osteotomy, whether done open or via minimally invasive technique, will allow the insertion point of the Achilles tendon to move upwards, simultaneously reducing the impingement at the retrocalcaneal bursa and giving a lengthening effect to the Achilles tendon

Pitfalls
- Focusing on only the tendon or the bone alone can lead to overlooking the true cause of the pathology and lead to recurrence
- Corticosteroid injections or surgical debridement of the distal end of the Achilles tendon alone can lead to its rupture.
- If greater than 30% of the Achilles tendon is detached, the surgeon is obliged to reinforce it at the time of surgery or risk complete rupture
- Calcaneoplasty alone without regard to pitch and morphology of the calcaneus may solve the initial retrocalcaneal impingement; however, it fails to address the overriding pathology and may leave the patient with achilles tightness, plantar fasciitis, and forefoot pain.

DISCLOSURE

The authors declare that they have no competing interests in the preparation or publication of this material.

REFERENCES

1. Ledoux WR, Shofer JB, Ahroni JH, et al. Biomechanical differences among pes cavus, neutrally aligned, and pes planus feet in subjects with diabetes. Foot Ankle Int 2003;24(11):845–50.
2. Aminian A, Sangeorzan BJ. The anatomy of cavus foot deformity. Foot Ankle Clin 2008;13(2):191–8, v.
3. Krähenbühl N, Weinberg MW. Anatomy and biomechanics of cavovarus deformity. Foot Ankle Clin 2019;24(2):173–81.
4. Tourné Y, Baray AL, Barthélémy R, et al. Contribution of a new radiologic calcaneal measurement to the treatment decision tree in Haglund syndrome. Orthopaedics & Traumatology, Surgery & Research : OTSR 2018;104(8):1215–9.
5. Tourne Y, Baray AL, Barthelemy R, et al. The Zadek calcaneal osteotomy in Haglund's syndrome of the heel: clinical results and a radiographic analysis to explain its efficacy. Foot Ankle Surg 2022;28(1):79–87.
6. Sella EJ, Caminear DS, McLarney EA. Haglund's syndrome. J Foot Ankle Surg 1998;37(2):110–4 [discussion: 173].
7. Stephens MM. Haglund's deformity and retrocalcaneal bursitis. Orthop Clin North Am 1994;25(1):41–6.
8. Easley ME, DeOrio MJ. Insertional achilles tendinopathy. In: Wiesel SW, Albert TJ, editors. Operative techniques in foot and ankle surgery. 3rd edition. Netherlands: Wolters Kluwer; 2022. p. 1193–202.
9. Kachlik D, Baca V, Cepelik M, et al. Clinical anatomy of the retrocalcaneal bursa. Surg Radiol Anat 2008;30(4):347–53.
10. Ahn JH, Ahn CY, Byun CH, et al. Operative treatment of haglund syndrome with central achilles tendon-splitting approach. J Foot Ankle Surg 2015;54(6):1053–6.

11. Thomas JL, Christensen JC, Kravitz SR, et al. The diagnosis and treatment of heel pain: a clinical practice guideline-revision 2010. J Foot Ankle Surg 2010;49(3 Suppl):S1–19.
12. Schepsis AA, Jones H, Haas AL. Achilles tendon disorders in athletes. Am J Sports Med 2002;30(2):287–305.
13. Uquillas CA, Guss MS, Ryan DJ, et al. Everything achilles: knowledge update and current concepts in management: AAOS exhibit selection. J Bone Joint Surg Am 2015;97(14):1187–95.
14. Holmes GB, Lin J. Etiologic factors associated with symptomatic achilles tendinopathy. Foot Ankle Int 2006;27(11):952–9.
15. Chinen T, Sasabuchi Y, Matsui H, et al. Association between third-generation fluoroquinolones and achilles tendon rupture: a self-controlled case series analysis. Ann Fam Med 2021;19(3):212–6.
16. Singh R, Rohilla R, Siwach RC, et al. Diagnostic significance of radiologic measurements in posterior heel pain. Foot 2008;18(2):91–8.
17. Wnuk-Scardaccione A, Mizia E, Zawojska K, et al. Surface shape of the calcaneal tuberosity and the occurrence of retrocalcaneal bursitis among runners. Int J Environ Res Publ Health 2021;18(6):2860.
18. Ruch JA. Haglund's disease. J Am Podiatry Assoc 1974;64(12):1000–3.
19. Heneghan MA, Pavlov H. The Haglund painful heel syndrome. Experimental investigation of cause and therapeutic implications. Clin Orthop Relat Res 1984;187:228–34.
20. Chauveaux D, Liet P, Le Huec JC, et al. A new radiologic measurement for the diagnosis of Haglund's deformity. Surg Radiol Anat 1991;13(1):39–44.
21. Lintz F, Mast J, Bernasconi A, et al. 3D, weightbearing topographical study of periprosthetic cysts and alignment in total ankle replacement. Foot Ankle Int 2020;41(1):1–9.
22. Lintz F, Ricard C, Mehdi N, et al. Hindfoot alignment assessment by the foot-ankle offset: a diagnostic study. Arch Orthop Trauma Surg 2023;143(5):2373–82.
23. Bernasconi A, Cooper L, Lyle S, et al. Intraobserver and interobserver reliability of cone beam weightbearing semi-automatic three-dimensional measurements in symptomatic pes cavovarus. Foot Ankle Surg 2020;26(5):564–72.
24. Lintz F, Jepsen M, De Cesar Netto C, et al. Distance mapping of the foot and ankle joints using weightbearing CT: The cavovarus configuration. Foot Ankle Surg 2021;27(4):412–20.
25. Covei-Banicioiu S, Ciurea PL, Parvanescu CD, et al. Ultrasonography role in evaluation of achilles tendon enthesis in reactive arthritis patients. Curr Health Sci J 2016;42(3):263–8.
26. Sundararajan PP, Wilde TS. Radiographic, clinical, and magnetic resonance imaging analysis of insertional Achilles tendinopathy. J Foot Ankle Surg 2014;53(2):147–51.
27. Krause F, Seidel A. Malalignment and lateral ankle instability: causes of failure from the varus tibia to the cavovarus foot. Foot Ankle Clin 2018;23(4):593–603.
28. Tourné Y, Mabit C, Moroney PJ, et al. Long-term follow-up of lateral reconstruction with extensor retinaculum flap for chronic ankle instability. Foot Ankle Int 2012;33(12):1079–86.
29. Wooten B, Uhl TL, Chandler J. Use of an orthotic device in the treatment of posterior heel pain. J Orthop Sports Phys Ther 1990;11(9):410–3.
30. Turmo-Garuz A, Rodas G, Balius R, et al. Can local corticosteroid injection in the retrocalcaneal bursa lead to rupture of the Achilles tendon and the medial head of the gastrocnemius muscle? Musculoskelet Surg 2014;98(2):121–6.

31. Vallone G, Vittorio T. Complete Achilles tendon rupture after local infiltration of corticosteroids in the treatment of deep retrocalcaneal bursitis. J Ultrasound 2014; 17(2):165–7.

32. Dean BJ, Lostis E, Oakley T, et al. The risks and benefits of glucocorticoid treatment for tendinopathy: a systematic review of the effects of local glucocorticoid on tendon. Semin Arthritis Rheum 2014;43(4):570–6.

33. Johannsen F, Olesen JL, Øhlenschläger TF, et al. Effect of ultrasonography-guided corticosteroid injection vs placebo added to exercise therapy for achilles tendinopathy: a randomized clinical trial. JAMA Netw Open 2022;5(7):e2219661.

34. Srivastava P, Aggarwal A. Ultrasound-guided retro-calcaneal bursa corticosteroid injection for refractory Achilles tendinitis in patients with seronegative spondyloarthropathy: efficacy and follow-up study. Rheumatol Int 2016;36(6):875–80.

35. O'Dowd A. Update on the Use of platelet-rich plasma injections in the management of musculoskeletal injuries: a systematic review of studies from 2014 to 2021. Orthop J Sports Med 2022;10(12). 23259671221140888.

36. van Sterkenburg MN, Muller B, Maas M, et al. Appearance of the weight-bearing lateral radiograph in retrocalcaneal bursitis. Acta Orthop 2010;81(3):387–90.

37. Checa A, Chun W, Pappu R. Ultrasound-guided diagnostic and therapeutic approach to Retrocalcaneal Bursitis. J Rheumatol 2011;38(2):391–2.

38. Boone SL, Uzor R, Walter E, et al. Safety and efficacy of image-guided retrocalcaneal bursa corticosteroid injection for the treatment of retrocalcaneal bursitis. Skeletal Radiol 2021;50(12):2471–82.

39. Chu NK, Lew HL, Chen CP. Ultrasound-guided injection treatment of retrocalcaneal bursitis. Am J Phys Med Rehabil 2012;91(7):635–7.

40. Goldberg-Stein S, Berko N, Thornhill B, et al. Fluoroscopically guided retrocalcaneal bursa steroid injection: description of the technique and pilot study of short-term patient outcomes. Skeletal Radiol 2016;45(8):1107–12.

41. Pi Y, Hu Y, Guo Q, et al. Calcaneoplasty coupled with an insertional Achilles tendon reattachment procedure for the prevention of secondary calcaneal impingement: a retrospective study. Ther Adv Chronic Dis 2020;11. 2040622320944793.

42. Alessio-Mazzola M, Russo A, Capello AG, et al. Endoscopic calcaneoplasty for the treatment of Haglund's deformity provides better clinical functional outcomes, lower complication rate, and shorter recovery time compared to open procedures: a systematic review. Knee Surg Sports Traumatol Arthrosc 2021;29(8): 2462–84.

43. Tourné Y, Francony F, Barthélémy R, et al. The Zadek calcaneal osteotomy in Haglund's syndrome of the heel: Its effects on the dorsiflexion of the ankle and correlations to clinical and functional scores. Foot Ankle Surg 2022;28(6):789–94.

44. Georgiannos D, Lampridis V, Vasiliadis A, et al. Treatment of insertional achilles pathology with dorsal wedge calcaneal osteotomy in athletes. Foot Ankle Int 2017;38(4):381–7.

45. López-Capdevila L, Santamaria Fumas A, Dominguez Sevilla A, et al. Dorsal wedge calcaneal osteotomy as surgical treatment for insertional Achilles tendinopathy. Rev Española Cirugía Ortopédica Traumatol 2020;64(1):22–7.

46. Maffulli N, Gougoulias N, D'Addona A, et al. Modified Zadek osteotomy without excision of the intratendinous calcific deposit is effective for the surgical treatment of calcific insertional Achilles tendinopathy. Surgeon 2021;19(6):e344–52.

47. Nordio A, Chan JJ, Guzman JZ, et al. Percutaneous Zadek osteotomy for the treatment of insertional Achilles tendinopathy. Foot Ankle Surg 2020;26(7): 818–21.

48. Vernois J, Redfern D, Ferraz L, et al. Minimally invasive surgery osteotomy of the hindfoot. Clin Podiatr Med Surg 2015;32(3):419–34.
49. Syed TA, Perera A. A proposed staging classification for minimally invasive management of haglund's syndrome with percutaneous and endoscopic surgery. Foot Ankle Clin 2016;21(3):641–64.
50. deMeireles AJ, Guzman JZ, Nordio A, et al. Complications after percutaneous osteotomies of the calcaneus. Foot Ankle Orthop 2022;7(3). 24730114221119731.
51. Malerba F, De Marchi F. Calcaneal osteotomies. Foot Ankle Clin 2005;10(3): 523–40, vii.
52. Chen J, Ramanathan D, Adams SB, et al. Midterm clinical and radiographic outcomes of the calcaneal Z-Osteotomy for the correction of cavovarus foot. Foot Ankle Orthop 2023;8(1). 24730114221146986.
53. Lohrer H. Minimum 3.5-year outcomes of operative treatment for Achilles tendon partial tears in the midportion and retrocalcaneal area. J Orthop Surg Res 2020; 15(1):395.
54. Lohrer H, Nauck T. Results of operative treatment for recalcitrant retrocalcaneal bursitis and midportion Achilles tendinopathy in athletes. Arch Orthop Trauma Surg 2014;134(8):1073–81.
55. Hardy A, Rousseau R, Issa SP, et al. Functional outcomes and return to sports after surgical treatment of insertional Achilles tendinopathy: Surgical approach tailored to the degree of tendon involvement. Orthopaedics & traumatology, surgery & research : OTSR 2018;104(5):719–23.
56. Lewis TL, Srirangarajan T, Patel A, et al. Clinical outcomes following surgical management of insertional Achilles tendinopathy using a double-row suture bridge technique with mean two-year follow-up. Eur J Orthop Surg Traumatol : Orthop Traumatol 2023;33(4):1179–84.
57. Güler Y, Birinci M, Hakyemez Ö S, et al. Achilles tendon-splitting approach and double-row suture anchor repair for Haglund syndrome. Foot Ankle Surg 2021; 27(4):421–6.
58. Lopes R, Padiolleau G, Fradet J, et al. Endoscopic SpeedBridge procedure for the treatment for insertional achilles tendinopathy: the snake technique. Arthrosc Tech 2021;10(9):e2127–34.
59. Howell MA, Catanzariti AR. Flexor hallucis longus tendon transfer for calcific insertional achilles tendinopathy. Clin Podiatr Med Surg 2016;33(1):113–23.
60. Howell MA, McConn TP, Saltrick KR, et al. Calcific insertional achilles tendinopathy-achilles repair with flexor hallucis longus tendon transfer: case series and surgical technique. J Foot Ankle Surg 2019;58(2):236–42.
61. Gamba C, Álvarez Gomez C, Martínez Zaragoza J, et al. Proximal medial gastrocnemius release: surgical technique. JBJS Essent Surg Tech 2022;12(1): e20.00039.
62. Barouk P. Technique, indications, and results of proximal medial gastrocnemius lengthening. Foot Ankle Clin 2014;19(4):795–806.

Midfoot Tarsectomy in Cavovarus: Why PSI Makes a Difference?

Julie Mathieu, MD[a], Louis Dagneaux, MD, PhD[a,b,*], CAOS France[c]

KEYWORDS

- Cavovarus deformity • Osteotomy • Patient-specific • 3D printing • Cutting guides
- Cavus

KEY POINTS

- The cavovarus foot is a complex and multiplanar foot deformity of the foot, that can be treated by anterior midfoot tarsectomy, which is a trapezoidal resection osteotomy with a dorsal base.
- While good functional results, this procedure was associated with substantial differences in the deformity correction and likely depending on the surgeon's experience.
- In addition to computer-assisted planning, patient-specific cutting guides (PSCGs) using 3D printing have shown many benefits in precision, reproducibility, ease to use, safety, reproducibility, and time savings when performing complex osteotomy.
- The use of PSCG to address multiplanar midfoot deformity is associated with improvements in accuracy and reliabililty from experimental results and clinical review.

Video content accompanies this article at http://www.foot.theclinics.com.

INTRODUCTION

Cavovarus foot is a multiplanar deformity of the forefoot, midfoot, and hindfoot combined, resulting in muscular imbalance. Excessive forefoot protonation leads to hindfoot varus compensation and external rotation of the leg axis during loading.[1]

[a] Department of Orthopedic Surgery, Lower Limb Surgery Unit, Univ Montpellier, 371 av. Gaston Giraud, Montpellier Cedex 05 34295, France; [b] Laboratoire de mécanique et génie civil (LMGC), CNRS, Montpellier University of Excellence (MUSE), 860, rue de St-Priest, Montpellier 34090, France; [c] CAOS (Computer Assisted Orthopaedic Surgery) France, Société Française de Chirurgie orthopédique et Traumatologie (SOFCOT), 56 Rue Boissonade, Paris 75014, France
* Corresponding author.
E-mail address: louisdagneaux@gmail.com

Foot Ankle Clin N Am 28 (2023) 791–803
https://doi.org/10.1016/j.fcl.2023.05.003
foot.theclinics.com

The surgical management of this debilitating condition involves several procedures ranging from isolated soft tissue procedures to triple arthrodesis.[2] Among the options available, anterior midfoot tarsectomy is indicated for moderate to severe deformities. The surgeon performs a trapezoidal resection osteotomy with a dorsal base at the midfoot, aiming to correct cavus and the excess forefoot protonation.[3]

While good functional results have been reported from international series, this technique remains difficult to perform with a limited margin of error[4,5]: the anterior tarsectomy must spare the Chopart's and Lisfranc's joints,[3] and appropriate correction of the deformity is the key. Overcorrection (leading to iatrogenic flatfoot) and undercorrection are both recognized as the risk for failures and dissatisfaction.[6] Finally, anterior midfoot tarsectomy is traditionally performed by a progressive, slow, and blind resection, which makes the appropriate correction difficult to achieve.

Over the past decade, the number of publications including patients treated by complex osteotomy using patient-specific instrumentation (PSI) and three-dimensional (3D) printed tools has increased in literature. Initially described in the context of osteotomies around the knee,[7] specific instrumentations have been utilized in various foot and ankle procedures, including total ankle replacements,[8,9] complex osteotomies[10,11] or tarsal coalition resection.[12] The benefits in using PSI are numerous: high accuracy,[13–16] increased intraoperative safety,[12,13,15] reduction in operating time and overall irradiation[9,12,13,15,16] cost-effectiveness,[9,12,13,15–17] decreased complications and revision rates, and increased functional outcomes.[18]

To date, two technical notes have been published regarding the use of PSCG in computer-assisted anterior midfoot tarsectomy[19,20] with limited follow-up and limited number of patients available. While these authors have reported good postoperative radiographic outcomes with no complications, the purpose of this article was to investigate and to discuss the role of PSCG in this procedure.

ANTERIOR MIDFOOT TARSECTOMY: PEARLS AND PITFALLS

Anterior midfoot tarsectomy, initially described by Sanders and Cole, is a multiplanar closed-wedge osteotomy performed at the apex of the deformity,[3] sparing the Chopart joint proximaly and the Lisfranc joint distally (**Fig. 1**). It thereby preserves the mobility of the hindfoot and forefoot. The objective of this trapezoidal resection is to normalize the Méary line and the Djian-Annonier angle.[5,21]

This is the most commonly performed midfoot osteotomy in literature when treating cavovarus foot, with a mean correction of 15° to 25° of the Djian-Annnonier angle.[6] Minimal resection in the cuboid does not, however, allow for the direct correction of forefoot adduction and some authors advise against it in cases of substantial adductus. However, the latter pitfall can be mitigate with careful preoperative planning: by

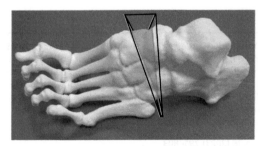

Fig. 1. Resection polyhedron related to the anterior midfoot tarsectomy, as described by Cole.

accentuating the dorsal resection at the intermediate cuneiform in order to increase the helical detorsion induced by the osteotomy.[4] Since tarsectomy can correct hindfoot varus and toe claws, some intraoperative adjustments and associated corrective procedures need to be made intraoperatively.

Our preference is to use two longitudinal approaches. The first, dorsomedial, is centered on the first or second metatarsal and allows access to the navicular and cuneiform. The second, dorsolateral approach is in line with the 4th metatarsal and allows access to the cuboid. In Cole's original technique, as reworked by Méary, the first cut made is the posterior one, which should be perpendicular to the hindfoot. It should spare the Chopart's joint and leave enough space on the cuboid and navicular to make place for the chosen osteosynthesis device[21] The distal cut was classically performed by careful removal with the gouge scissors by Méary, allowing for progressive correction. Like the first cut, it must leave enough space on the dorsal surfaces of the cuneiform and cuboid to allow internal fixation.[3,21]

Immobilization with a short leg cast was performed with no weightbearing for 9 to 12 weeks. After this period, patients were allowed to walk as tolerated, depending on residual pain and swelling.

Some case series have been published in the last two-decades, aiming to report the clinical and radiographic outcomes of the conventional technique (**Table 1**). These series included a limited number of patients (mean of 20, ranging from 3 to 52), with variable follow-up[2,4,5,22–26] Overall, better radiographic outcomes were reported in reducible deformity[4,5] and all series have shown improvements in pain, function, gait pattern, hyper-pressure, and hyperkeratosis phenomena, and overall patient satisfaction.[2,22–26]

However, the authors highlighted the risk for the variable correction of the deformity using the freehand technique, and some intraoperative complications have been reported, including fracture of the midfoot bones or excessive resection.[5] Undercorrection and overcorrection are both recognized factors leading to failure: iatrogenic flatfoot, residual deformity, recurrence, and ultimately, adverse functional outcomes.[1–3,27] In particular, Jarde and colleagues found that undercorrection may resulted in recurrence, pain, and dissatisfaction.[22] While the restoration of the Méary line remains a reliable prognostic factor,[5] under-correction rates up to 80% of the cases[5] and iatrogenic flatfoot up to 23%[4] in some series. In addition, while good mean correction was usually reported in the literature, postoperative Meary's angle ranged from −21° to 35° (see **Table 1**). Anterior tarsectomy is therefore effective, but it relies on the surgeon's experience to determine the correct amount of bone to resect, intraoperatively.

3D PRINTING AND PATIENT-SPECIFIC INSTRUMENTATION

Since specific instrumentation has been developed for computer-assisted osteotomies around the knee, their use in foot and ankle surgery is currently the subject of numerous publications. The main advance from patient-specific cutting guides is related to tumor resection,[28] where the success of the surgical procedure depends on the accuracy of the correction or removal. In this particular context, the authors have found more resections in healthy margins,[29] less recurrence at the last follow-up[30] no intraoperative soft tissue lesions[29,30] and results that may be identical between experienced and novice surgeons.[29] In foot and ankle surgery, the main publications about 3D printing and PSI concerned the implantation of total ankle replacements, since implants survival relies on implants positioning more than any other total joint replacement.[14,31] Other indications have been found: surgical management of calcaneus fractures,[32] removal of

Table 1
Recent literature review about anterior midfoot tarsectomy

Authors	Study Type	N (Feet)	Mean Age	Mean Follow-up	Postoperative Meary Angle (Mean, Range)	Postoperative Djian-Annonier Angle (Mean, Range)	Postoperative AOFAS Score	Specific Postoperative Complications
Jarde et al,[22] 2001	Retrospective	52	40	6.5y	8°	125° (N/A)	-	Undercorrection (21%), overcorrection (6%)
Tullis et al,[25] 2004	Retrospective	10	N/A	23m	-	-	-	Toe claws recurrence (1 case)
Sraj et al,[2] 2008	Retrospective	5	20	13y	5.7° (N/A)	-	-	Cavus recurrence (1 case)
Johnson et al,[23] 2009	Retrospective	3	25	1y	5.6° (4 – 8)	-	-	-
Naudi et al,[5] 2009	Retrospective	39	31	9.8y	9° (-6 – 35)	111.3° (92 – 134)	69.2	Partial nonunion (1 case), overcorrection (2 cases), undercorrection (1 case), cavus recurrence (1 case)
Zhou et al,[26]	Prospective	17	N/A	25.3m	5.5° (N/A)	-	75.8	-
Simon et al,[4]	Retrospective	26	16	6.2y	-1.4° (-21 – 20)	-	95.5	Overcorrection (23%)
Ergun & Yildirim,[24] 2019	Retrospective	6	22	15.3m	8.7	-	79.5	Partial nonunion (1 case)

Abbreviations: AOFAS, American Orthopaedic Foot & Ankle Society; m, month; N, number; N/A, non available; y, year.

intraosseous cysts,[15] ligamentoplasty[16] subtalar arthrodesis[13] or resections of tarsal coalitions finally corresponding to multiplanar osteotomies.[12] As such, the benefits of custom instrumentation and 3D printing are found in numerous publications on foot and ankle surgery: increased precision,[12,14,16,29,33,34] facilitation of the operative procedure and diffusion of complex techniques to untrained surgeons,[12,15,29] intraoperative safety,[9,12,13,15,29,32] reduction in operating time,[9,12,13,16,29] and decrease in radiation exposure.[9,12,13,16,29] Therefore, all these advantages should profit to other complex procedures, namely anterior midfoot tarsectomy.

COMPUTER-ASSISTED ANTERIOR TARSECTOMY

Two studies using PSCG applied to anterior tarsectomy have been published, both technical notes with good postoperative radiographic results.[19,20] We described the original technique in 2019 in the Foot and Ankle International journal.[19] We used a polyamide 2200 patient-specific cutting guide with sawblade windows, in contrast with the more recent technique published by Sobrón and colleagues In this technique, they used 2 custom-made guides made of thermoplastic acid (PLA) for the positioning of 1.5 mm Kirshner wires; these wires secondarily guided the saw blade allowing the osteotomy to be completed with the osteotome on the medial and lateral sides of the midfoot.[20] In both cases, the planned correction was determined from weight-bearing radiographs and then transferred to the 3D models from CT-scan using dedicated software.

In our technique, Bone geometries were extracted from preoperative CT-scan slices (GE LightSpeed VCT64) according to the following protocol: identical coordinate system and Field Of View at 35 for all acquisitions, voltage at 120 kV, current at 400 mA, 512x512 matrix, constant pixel size throughout the examination. Acquisitions started at least 5 cm above the talocrural joint and included the entire foot up to the toes. The slice thickness was set at 0.625 mm in bone filter. Then, computer-assisted design (CAD) software was used to obtain patient-specific 3D model by automatic segmentation (Simpleware computer software; Synopsys, Mountain View, CA). This 3D model allowed us to understand the complexity of the cavovarus deformity, and to plan appropriate correction from the angular measures performed on radiographs. Therefore, the resection polyhedron (location and volume) and the correction of the deformity after closed wedge osteotomy were simulated on the 3D model using Creo Parametric software (PTC Boston, MA) (**Fig. 2**). In this step, closed collaboration between surgeon and engineer is the key.

After surgical validation, a patient and deformity-specific cutting guide was simulated and printed in polyamide PA 2200 (EOS GmbH-Electro Optical Systems, Munich, Germany). The guide was then sterilized (270°F; exposure time, 4 minutes; drying time, 20 minutes) to follow operating room recommendations. Finally, a 3D foot model before and after correction was also printed and sterilized in the same way to allow the surgeon, intraoperatively, to visualize the correction and the remaining bone surfaces for optimizing internal fixation (**Fig. 3**). The specifications for each guide had to meet the following conditions, according to the original technique[19].

- To perform an anterior tarsectomy sparing the Chopart (calcaneo-cuboid and talo-navicular) and Lisfranc joints and correcting the Méary line and the Djian-Annonier angle.
- The resection had to be dorsally based wedge-shaped, narrower externally in the cuboid, and with sufficient space within the navicular, cuboid, and cuneiforms to allow for osteosynthesis.

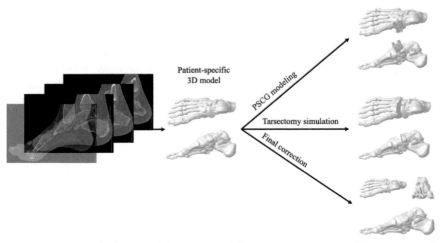

Fig. 2. Patient-specific foot model was created from CT-scan images, with cutting guide modeling and simulation of the closed-wedge osteotomy.

- The orientation of the Kirshner wires allowing the positioning of the guide had to protect the dorsal and plantar structures by constraining the movements of the saw blade (**Fig. 4**).

Regarding our surgical technique, the patient-specific cutting guide was applied via a medial longitudinal approach of approximately 6 to 7 cm (**Fig. 5**) and fixed with 2.2 mm Kirshner wires from pins area provided for this purpose, once perfect congruence was obtained between the jig, the navicular, and the first two cuneiforms. The residual length of the wires outside the guide was determined by 3D planning, avoiding

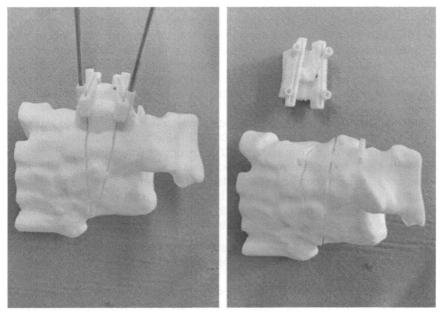

Fig. 3. 3D printed foot with planed bone cuts and dedicated cutting jig.

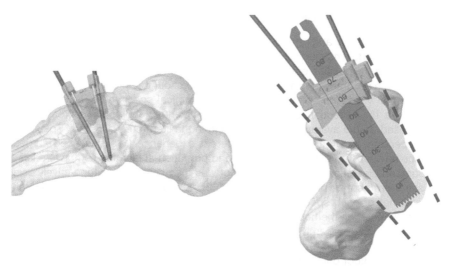

Fig. 4. Osteotomy corridor with respect to the k-wires orientation.

soft-tissue injuries (in particular, lateral pinning of the short fibular tendon or plantar effraction). Additionally, a lateral approach centered on the cuboid was then performed to control wire positioning from the lateral side of the midfoot. The osteotomy was then performed through the sawblade window using a precision sawblade (Precision FALCON Oscillating Tip Saw, Stryker, USA), and the closed-wedge effect was performed manually by plantar deflection (Video 1 – supplemental) and fixed with staples and locking plates. Intraoperative radiographs and computer model were available in the operating room to ensure the concordance between the theoretical planning and the practical reality.

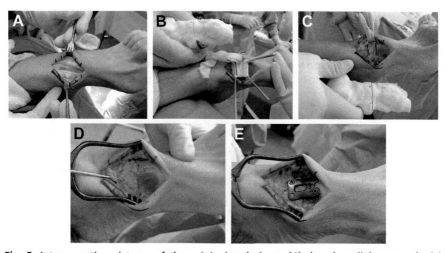

Fig. 5. Intraoperative pictures of the original technique: (A) dorsal-medial approach, (B) positioning of the cutting guide fixed with 2.2 mm K wires, (C) bone cuts in accordance with 3D printed object, (D) osteotomy closure fixed with temporary pins, (E) internal fixation with unspecific locking plate.

EXPERIMENTAL VALIDATION

Overall, the accuracy and reproducibility of 3D printed objects should use pre-clinical analysis (eg, cadaveric studies) or computed post-hoc analysis to investigate the variability around the position of the 3D object or the error of instrumentation trajectories. To ensure the accuracy, reproducibility, and safety of our technique, we conducted an experimental validation study, including 10 anatomical specimens. Using the same workflow, a 15° correction of the Méary line was planned and applied on each specimen, based on the average resections found in the literature.[2,4,5,22,23,35] Specimens were operated on by 2 operators of different experience (1 experienced surgeon and one novice). The osteotomy closure and pronation-supination setup were left at the surgeon discretion. Each operated foot was then scanned postoperatively using the same protocol as previously described. 3D reconstruction in stereo-lithography (STL) format of each specimen was modeled with a dedicated software using the same segmentation method and postoperative 3D reconstruction was compared to 3D planning using a semi-automatic matching process already described in other publication[28,36–38] **(Fig. 6)**. In this step, we only focused on differences (postop. vs planned) in midfoot bones (cuboid, navicular, and cuneiforms), using Mesh software (CloudCompare, EDF, R&D, Paris, France), and angular deviations were evaluated using transformation matrices with CAD software (PTC Creo, Boston, Massachusetts, USA). Finally, the safety of the procedure was assessed by secondary dissections verifying the absence of tendon or neurovascular injury.

In this experimental study, we found a very good accuracy with limited error of mapping distance between postoperative and planned models (mean of 1.6; CI95%: 1.2–2.0 mm), with 92% of the surfaces were within 2 mm of the planning with a Gaussian distribution (see **Fig. 6**). The closed-wedge accuracy in the sagittal plane was of 2° (95% CI: 1.4° – 3.6°), with no significant difference between operators. After the dissection of the specimens, no tendon or neurovascular lesions were found. As such, these preliminary results tent to confirm better accuracy and reliability among operators with computer-assisted technique and patient-specific cutting guides in comparison with freehanded technique reported in historical literature.

CLINICAL VALIDATION

From January 2019 and January 2022, 10 patients with cavovarus foot were eligible for anterior midfoot tarsectomy and operated on in our department. In this retrospective study, cavovarus deformity was neurological in 50%, post-traumatic in 25%, and

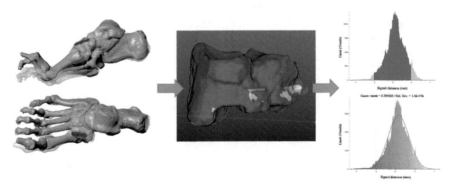

Fig. 6. 3D mapping showing the point-to-surface distances within 2 mm of plan. Corresponding histogram and gauss repartition centered around 0 mm.

idiopathic in 25%. Mean follow-up was 15.3 months [3–42 months]. The surgical procedure was the same as the one previously described, but with the addition of a reduction guide to assist pronation-supination setup. Four patients benefited from additional procedures, including 4 calcaneal osteotomies and 1 additional dorsal-based closed wedge osteotomy of the first metatarsal. Clinical results using AOFAS score and radiographic outcomes from weight-bearing radiographs were assessed, as well as the occurrence of postoperative complications.

The AOFAS midfoot score significantly improved by 45 ± 21 points for a mean postoperative score of 73 ± 24 ($P = .001$) and the VAS improved by 4 ± 3 points for a mean postoperative VAS of 2 ± 3 ($P = .007$). Regarding the radiographic outcomes, the Méary line was restored with a mean postoperative angle of 2° ± 3° (**Fig. 7**). Similarly, the postoperative Djian-Annonier angle was considered as normalized in most of the cases, with a mean angle of 120° (SD, 6.6°). Postoperative complications were dominated by 2 partial non-unions involving the medial naviculo-cuneal arthrodesis, one of which was completely asymptomatic.

DISCUSSION

The complexity of the cavovarus foot deformity makes the execution of a multiplanar resection difficult to achieve using the freehand technique. In this context, patient-specific instrumentation may allow precise bone resection to address the desired surgical correction, even in the hands of an untrained operator, with safety improvements in regards to soft tissues and surrounding joints. Secondary, the preoperative 3D modeling allows for a better understanding of the deformity and its correction.

With respect to our experimental validation and clinical review, accuracy in targeting a normal Méary's line was excellent, both in vitro and in vivo. These preliminary results confirm the precision and reproducibility of computer-assisted anterior midfoot tarsectomy. The main clinical relevance of this new technology is to minimize the risk for angular error, which is the main cause of failure of this procedure. While previous

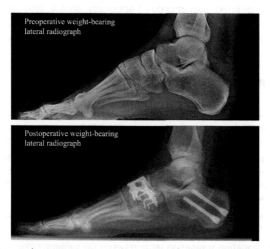

Fig. 7. Preoperative and postoperative radiographs of a 43-year-old man who underwent computer-assisted anterior tarsectomy with cutting guide, and an additional Zadek-type calcaneal osteotomy. Radiographs showed a normalized Méary line (from 15° to 0°) and a corrected Djian-Annonier angle (from 112.7° to 125.5°).

studies have found particularly high undercorrection[5] and overcorrection rate https://www.deepl.com/translator?utm_source = windows&utm_medium = app&utm_campaign = windows-shares,[4] we did not find such outliers from our experimental and clinical investigations.

While angular correction was planned from conventional weight-bearing radiographs in our technique, the asset of modern 3D imaging modalities such as WBCT in the understanding of cavovarus deformity in weight-bearing conditions and targeting the "true" 3D correction. The main limitation remains in the creation of the cutting guides from WBCT images since patients are positioned supine in the operating room. Weight-bearing and non-weight-bearing conditions can change the interaction between midfoot bones, and therefore, limit the capability of the cutting jig to fit with bones contours intraoperatively.

Industrial considerations and team workflow between surgeons and engineers are of primary importance. The position, orientation, and dimensions of the saw window may improve the safety of this procedure, reducing the risk for the sawblade to slipe out the osteotomy corridor (oriented in lateral and plantar). 3d printed reduction jig could be implemented in the original technique to assist the surgeon in the reduction of the osteotomy and pronation-supination setup. Importantly, the use of an oscillating tip saw is highly recommended when using cutting jigs, to reduce saw binding within the saw window. To date, little is known about the role of debris generation on nonunion occurrence and therefore, the use of house-made jigs with unvalidated biomaterials should be considered with extreme caution.

Lastly, the need for patient-specific internal fixation methods should be considered to improve outcomes and decrease the risk for non-union. In particular, patient-specific implants with 3D printed locking plates may represent an additional step in this patient-specific strategy.

SUMMARY

While anterior midfoot tarsectomy is a complex procedure with a substantial risk for complications and failures, computer-assisted procedure with patient-specific cutting guides seemed associated with improved accuracy, safety, and reliability among operators. The advantages of patient-specific instrumentation should not obviate the importance of concomitant bone and soft-tissue procedures when treating severe cavovarus foot.

CLINICS CARE POINTS

- Anterior midfoot tarsectomy, is a multiplanar closed-wedge osteotomy performed at the apex of the deformity, that must spare the Chopart and the Lisfranc joints.
- The objective of this trapezoidal resection is to normalize the Méary's line and the Djian-Annonier's angle. While good outcomes are generally reported from limited cases-series, free-handed conventional technique is associated with high rates of undercorrection and iatrogenic flatfoot.
- Computer-assisted planning, in association with patient-specific instrumentation, are associated with high reliability for restoring the Meary's line.
- After resection, pronation-supination setup relies on the surgeon's experience, disregarding the patient-specific instrumentation.
- The need for patient-specific internal fixation methods should be considered to decrease the risk for non-union, while remaining rare.

- The advantages of patient-specific instrumentation should not obviate the importance of concomitant bone and soft-tissue procedures when treating severe cavovarus foot.

DECLARATION OF CONFLICTING INTERESTS

One of the authors declared potential conflicts of interest with respect to the research, authorship, and/or publication of this article. ICMJE forms for all authors are available online.

FUNDING

The author(s) received no financial support for the research, authorship, and/or publication of this article.

ETHICAL REVIEW COMMITTEE

Each author certifies that his institution has approved the reporting of these cases and that all investigations were conducted in conformity with the ethical principles of research.

DISCLOSURE

Dr L. Dagneaux reports grants and personal fees from Newclip Technics, during the conduct of the study; grants from Société Française de Chirurgie orthopédique et Traumatologie (SOFCOT), France, grants from University of Montpellier, France, grants from University Hospital of Montpellier, personal fees from Newclip Technics, personal fees from Zimmer biomet, personal fees from Depuy Synthes, research grants from Exatech, research grants from Labex Numev, outside the submitted work.

ACKNOWLEDGMENTS

The authors are indebted of Guillaume Lamouroux (Newclip techniques) for his support.

SUPPLEMENTARY DATA

Supplementary data related to this article can be found online at https://doi.org/10.1016/j.fcl.2023.05.003.

REFERENCES

1. Wicart P. Cavus foot, from neonates to adolescents. Orthop Traumatol Surg Res 2012;98(7):813–28.
2. Sraj SA, Saghieh S, Abdulmassih S, et al. Medium to Long-term Follow-up Following Correction of Pes Cavus Deformity. J Foot Ankle Surg 2008;47(6):527–32.
3. MEARY R, MATTEI CR, TOMENO B. Tarsectomie anterieure pour pied creux. indications et resultats lointainS. Tarsectomie anterieure pour pied creux indic result lointains 1976;62(2):231–43.
4. Simon AL, Seringe R, Badina A, et al. Long term results of the revisited Meary closing wedge tarsectomy for the treatment of the fixed cavo-varus foot in adolescent with Charcot-Marie-Tooth disease. Foot Ankle Surg 2019;25(6):834–41.

5. Naudi S, Dauplat G, Staquet V, et al. Anterior tarsectomy long-term results in adult pes cavus. Orthop Traumatol Surg Res 2009;95(4):293–300.

6. Maynou C, Szymanski C, Thiounn A. The adult cavus foot. EFORT Open Rev 2017;2(5):221–9.

7. Munier M, Donnez M, Ollivier M, et al. Can three-dimensional patient-specific cutting guides be used to achieve optimal correction for high tibial osteotomy? Pilot study. Orthop Traumatol Surg Res 2017;103(2):245–50.

8. Daigre J, Berlet G, Van Dyke B, et al. Accuracy and Reproducibility Using Patient-Specific Instrumentation in Total Ankle Arthroplasty. Foot Ankle Int 2017;38(4):412–8.

9. Saito GH, Sanders AE, O'Malley MJ, et al. Accuracy of patient-specific instrumentation in total ankle arthroplasty: A comparative study. Foot Ankle Surg 2019;25(3):383–9.

10. Lachman JR, Adams SB. Tibiotalocalcaneal Arthrodesis for Severe Talar Avascular Necrosis. Foot Ankle Clin 2019;24(1):143–61.

11. Giovinco NA, Dunn SP, Dowling L, et al. A Novel Combination of Printed 3-Dimensional Anatomic Templates and Computer-assisted Surgical Simulation for Virtual Preoperative Planning in Charcot Foot Reconstruction. J Foot Ankle Surg 2012;51(3):387–93.

12. Sobrón FB, Benjumea A, Alonso MB, et al. 3D Printing Surgical Guide for Talocalcaneal Coalition Resection: Technique Tip. Foot Ankle Int 2019;40(6):727–32.

13. Duan XJ, Fan HQ, Wang FY, et al. Application of 3D-printed Customized Guides in Subtalar Joint Arthrodesis. Orthop Surg 2019;11(3):405–13.

14. Berlet GC, Penner MJ, Lancianese S, et al. Total Ankle Arthroplasty Accuracy and Reproducibility Using Preoperative CT Scan-Derived, Patient-Specific Guides. Foot Ankle Int 2014;35(7):665–76.

15. Zhang C, Cao J, Zhu H, et al. Endoscopic Treatment of Symptomatic Foot and Ankle Bone Cyst with 3D Printing Application. BioMed Res Int 2020;2020. https://doi.org/10.1155/2020/8323658.

16. Wu Q, Yu T, Lei B, et al. A New Individualized Three-Dimensional Printed Template for Lateral Ankle Ligament Reconstruction. Med Sci Monit Int Med J Exp Clin Res 2020;26. e922925-1-e922925-7.

17. Hamid KS, Matson AP, Nwachukwu BU, et al. Determining the Cost-Savings Threshold and Alignment Accuracy of Patient-Specific Instrumentation in Total Ankle Replacements. Foot Ankle Int 2017;38(1):49–57.

18. de Wouters S, Tran Duy K, Docquier PL. Patient-specific instruments for surgical resection of painful tarsal coalition in adolescents. Orthop Traumatol Surg Res 2014;100(4):423–7.

19. Dagneaux L, Canovas F. 3D Printed Patient-Specific Cutting Guide for Anterior Midfoot Tarsectomy. Foot Ankle Int 2020;41(2):211–5.

20. Sobrón FB, Dos Santos-Vaquinhas A, Alonso B, et al. Technique tip: 3D printing surgical guide for pes cavus midfoot osteotomy. Foot Ankle Surg 2021. https://doi.org/10.1016/j.fas.2021.05.001. S1268773121000904.

21. Cole WH. The classic. The treatment of claw-foot. By Wallace H. Cole. 1940. Clin Orthop 1983;(181):3–6.

22. Jarde O, Abi Raad G, Vernois J, et al. Tarsectomie antérieure pour pied creux essentiel. Etude rétrospective de 52 cas [Anterior tarsectomy for cavus foot. Retrospective study of 52 cases]. Acta Orthop Belg 2001;67(5):481–7.

23. Johnson BM, Child B, Hix J, et al. Cavus Foot Reconstruction in 3 Patients with Charcot-Marie-Tooth Disease. J Foot Ankle Surg 2009;48(2):116–24.

24. Ergun S, Yildirim Y. The Cole Midfoot Osteotomy: Clinical and Radiographic Retrospective Review of Five Patients (Six Feet) with Different Etiologies. J Am Podiatr Med Assoc 2019;109(3):180–6.

25. Tullis BL, Mendicino RW, Catanzariti AR, et al. The Cole midfoot osteotomy: a retrospective review of 11 procedures in 8 patients. J Foot Ankle Surg Off Publ Am Coll Foot Ankle Surg 2004;43(3):160–5.

26. Zhou Y, Zhou B, Liu J, et al. A prospective study of midfoot osteotomy combined with adjacent joint sparing internal fixation in treatment of rigid pes cavus deformity. J Orthop Surg 2014;9:44. https://doi.org/10.1186/1749-799X-9-44.

27. Mestdagh H, Maynou C, Butin E, et al. Pes cavus in the adult. In: Bouysset M, editor. Bone and joint disorders of the foot and ankle. Deutschland: Springer Berlin Heidelberg; 1998. p. 173–82. https://doi.org/10.1007/978-3-662-06132-9_16.

28. Jud L, Müller DA, Fürnstahl P, et al. Joint-preserving tumour resection around the knee with allograft reconstruction using three-dimensional preoperative planning and patient-specific instruments. Knee 2019;26(3):787–93.

29. Cartiaux O, Paul L, Francq BG, et al. Improved accuracy with 3D planning and patient-specific instruments during simulated pelvic bone tumor surgery. Ann Biomed Eng 2014;42(1):205–13.

30. Cernat E, Docquier PL, Paul L, et al. Patient Specific Instruments for Complex Tumor Resection-Reconstruction Surgery within the Pelvis: A Series of 4 Cases. Chir Buchar Rom 1990 2016;111(5):439–44.

31. Dagneaux L, Nogue E, Mathieu J, et al. Survivorship of 4,748 Contemporary Total Ankle Replacements from the French Discharge Records Database. J Bone Jt Surg 2022. https://doi.org/10.2106/JBJS.21.00746.

32. Wang C, Xu C, Li M, et al. Patient-specific instrument-assisted minimally invasive internal fixation of calcaneal fracture for rapid and accurate execution of a preoperative plan: A retrospective study. BMC Muscoskel Disord 2020;21. https://doi.org/10.1186/s12891-020-03439-3.

33. Zhang YW, Xiao X, Xiao Y, et al. Efficacy and Prognosis of 3D Printing Technology in Treatment of High-Energy Trans-Syndesmotic Ankle Fracture Dislocation - "Log-Splitter" Injury. Med Sci Monit Int Med J Exp Clin Res 2019;25:4233–43.

34. Wu M, Guan J, Xiao Y, et al. Application of three-dimensional printing technology for closed reduction and percutaneous cannulated screws fixation of displaced intraarticular calcaneus fractures. Zhongguo Xiu Fu Chong Jian Wai Ke Za Zhi Zhongguo Xiufu Chongjian Waike Zazhi Chin J Reparative Reconstr Surg 2017; 31(11):1316–21.

35. Hewitt SM, Tagoe M. Surgical Management of Pes Cavus Deformity with an Underlying Neurological Disorder: A Case Presentation. J Foot Ankle Surg 2011; 50(2):235–40.

36. Vlachopoulos L, Schweizer A, Graf M, et al. Three-dimensional postoperative accuracy of extra-articular forearm osteotomies using CT-scan based patient-specific surgical guides. BMC Muscoskel Disord 2015;16. https://doi.org/10.1186/s12891-015-0793-x.

37. Gouin F, Paul L, Odri GA, et al. Computer-Assisted Planning and Patient-Specific Instruments for Bone Tumor Resection within the Pelvis: A Series of 11 Patients. Sarcoma 2014;1–9.

38. Müller DA, Stutz Y, Vlachopoulos L, et al. The Accuracy of Three-Dimensional Planned Bone Tumor Resection Using Patient-Specific Instrument. Cancer Manag Res 2020;12:6533–40.

Hindfoot Fusions in the Cavovarus Foot

What Is the Key for a Successful Outcome?

Matthew James Welck, MBBS, BSc, MSc, FRCS(Orth)*,
Anil Haldar, MBBS, FRCS (Orth)

KEYWORDS

- Cavovarus foot • Cavus • Arthrodesis • Triple fusion • Tendon transfer
- Wedge tarsectomy

KEY POINTS

- The aim of surgical management is to establish a painless, plantigrade, balanced and stable foot.
- A comprehensive clinical and radiographic assessment enables the surgeon to fully understand the patient's deformity and plan a reliable surgical strategy for deformity correction.
- Rigid deformities should be corrected at their apex either in the hindfoot or midfoot.
- Surgical correction must include tendon transfers when required to balance the soft tissues to reduce the risk of deformity recurrence in the long-term.

INTRODUCTION

The cavovarus foot deformity can vary in severity from subtle and flexible to severe and rigid.[1]

Treatment options for the cavovarus foot include non-operative measures such as shoe-wear modification, custom orthotics and analgesics. Orthotics aim to realign a flexible hindfoot deformity or to accommodate and distribute the pressure of a fixed hindfoot deformity.[1–3] When these simple measures fail, patients may progress to surgical intervention.

The aim of surgical management is to establish a painless, plantigrade, balanced and stable foot.[1,2] In the case of subtle or flexible deformities, this goal can often be achieved with a combination of soft tissue release or lengthening, joint sparing hindfoot, midfoot or forefoot osteotomies and tendon transfers.[1–3]

Department of Foot and Ankle Surgery, Royal National Orthopaedic Hospital, London, UK
* Corresponding author. Foot and Ankle Unit, Royal National Orthopadic NHS Trust, Brockley Hill, Stanmore, HA7 4LP, UK.
E-mail address: matthewwelck@doctors.org.uk

Foot Ankle Clin N Am 28 (2023) 805–818
https://doi.org/10.1016/j.fcl.2023.05.004
1083-7515/23/Crown Copyright © 2023 Published by Elsevier Inc. All rights reserved.

foot.theclinics.com

In patients with rigid deformities and those with established articular degenerative change, joint sparing techniques are less likely to be successful.[3,4] In such circumstances, hindfoot fusions are often required to achieve the goals of surgery.[1-5] The objective of this article is to outline the key for a successful outcome when performing hindfoot fusions in the cavovarus foot.

TYPES OF CAVUS DEFORMITY

The first step to achieving a successful outcome in managing the cavus foot is to understand the patient's deformity, in order to formulate a reliable surgical strategy. We will explore these deformities in turn, explaining salient features to evaluate clinically and go on to consider the impact these findings have on achieving a successful surgical outcome.

The cavus foot is defined as a foot with a high medial arch.[2] This high arch rarely occurs in isolation and four common patterns of cavus foot deformity are recognised: the "pure" cavus foot, the cavovarus foot, the equinocavovarus foot and the calcaneocavus foot.[6]

The pure cavus foot can be idiopathic in nature or secondary to neurological causes. It is characterised by an increased medial arch alone with no other associated deformities.

A cavovarus deformity is more common and results from muscular imbalance with weakness of eversion when compared to inversion. The most common cause of this is Charcot-Marie-Tooth (CMT) disease, which results in weakness of tibialis anterior and peroneus brevis when compared to tibialis posterior and peroneus longus. The resultant deformity is a foot drop coupled with hindfoot varus and forefoot pronation. There are also often claw toes, which occur due to extensor substitution, where the long toe extensors try to compensate for weak dorsiflexion of the ankle caused by tibialis anterior weakness. Hyperextension occurs at the metatarsophalangeal joints of the lesser toes and the long toe flexors pull the distal phalanges into plantar flexion leading to clawing.

An equinocavovarus foot occurs most commonly secondary to neurological causes such as cerebral palsy, hereditary spastic paraplegia, stroke or post-compartment syndrome[6,7] (**Fig. 1**). Patients with a residual congenital talipes equinovarus deformity would also typically display this deformity. It is normally driven by spasticity and relative overactivity of the calf muscles compared to the ankle dorsiflexors, leading to foot equinus and plantarflexion of the forefoot, especially the first ray due to excessive peroneus longus contraction. First ray plantarflexion causes a compensatory foot cavus and heel varus alongside the equinus deformity.[6]

The calcaneocavus deformity occurs due to muscular imbalance between ankle dorsiflexors and plantarflexors, resulting in dorsiflexion of the hindfoot and compensatory forefoot plantarflexion. Causes of this can again be neurological such as cerebral palsy and myelomeningocoele. Another scenario where this is seen is iatrogenic overlengthening of the Achilles tendon, leading to an increased calcaneal pitch angle on lateral radiographic imaging and a cavus foot.[6]

Recognising the specific type of cavus deformity, with an appreciation of the underlying pathogenesis, is crucial to understanding and therefore appropriately planning deformity correction surgery. There can be no standard algorithm for these complex deformities and each patient must be judged on their own merit, bearing these patterns in mind.

EVALUATING CAVUS DEFORMITIES AND MUSCLE BALANCE

Patients must be clinically assessed by taking a comprehensive history, acknowledging comorbidities such as neurological issues and previous surgery. Certain neurological conditions are associated with typical patterns of deformity.

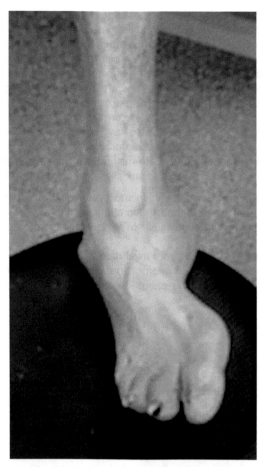

Fig. 1. Clinical photograph of a rigid equinocavovarus deformity.

The specific foot and ankle examination should include an assessment of the patient's footwear and gait. Global inspection of the feet can reveal the cavus foot deformity type and identify hindfoot, midfoot and forefoot deformity components and signs of pressure areas. Tenderness should be elicited by systematic palpation of the feet and mobility of deformities should be established, understanding if the cavus foot is flexible and correctible or rigid and stiff. First ray mobility should also be noted.[1–3]

The Coleman Block test can be helpful in assessing correctability of the hindfoot, however simple assessment of the movement of the subtalar joint with the patient non-weightbearing also serves as a useful guide to whether the hindfoot deformity is rigid or flexible.[4,5] The Silfverskiold test is essential to assess if the Achilles tendon is contracted or if the gastrocnemius is tight. Achilles lengthening or gastrocnemius recession may then be planned as part of deformity correction surgery based on this assessment. The relaxation of a gastrocnemius contracture may also induce some flexibility in a seemingly rigid deformity.

A full systemic, local and neurological examination should be performed, assessing for possible spinal or neurological etiologies for the cavus foot deformity.[2] It is imperative to evaluate muscle power, commonly using the Medical Research Council (MRC) power scale.[1,2,4] Specifically, the major hindfoot invertor, tibialis posterior, must be compared to peroneus brevis and longus as these muscles may be causing the cavovarus foot deformity and often need to be transferred as part of corrective surgery.[8] Furthermore, power of ankle dorsiflexion and plantarflexion should be assessed, as for example, a foot drop may have bearing on choice of tendon transfer.

Relevant imaging is also essential for surgical planning. Plain weight-bearing AP and lateral radiographs of both ankles and a dorsoplantar weight-bearing view of both feet should be obtained to identify the site of deformity and also the degree of correction that may be required.[1,2] In our unit, we also have access to weight-bearing computed tomography (CT), which has proved a helpful and informative tool in understanding these complex multiplanar deformity patterns and helps us to plan accurate correction surgery (**Fig. 2**). It is important to systematically appreciate the deformity at all levels.

- *Ankle*: Evaluate for varus at the ankle and if present, whether joint is congruent or incongruent. Also evaluate for arthritic changes.
- *Hindfoot*: Evaluate for talonavicular over coverage, hindfoot varus, evidence of arthritis.
- *Midfoot*: Evaluate for sagittal and axial deformity in the midfoot. For example, is there adduction through the midfoot that might persist after correction of the hindfoot? Is the apex of the cavus deformity in the midfoot, rather than the hindfoot?

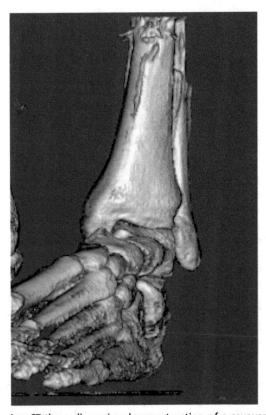

Fig. 2. Weight-bearing CT three-dimensional reconstruction of a cavovarus foot.

- *Forefoot*: Evaluate for first metatarsal pronation, or pronation of the entire fore-foot. Metatarsus adductus. Toe deformities.

In our unit, the CT scans can also be used to inform custom patient specific cutting guides to permit accurate planning and deformity correction surgery in specific types of deformity.[9,10]

PLANNING AND PERFORMING CAVUS HINDFOOT CORRECTION SURGERY

Once the information regarding the patient's cavus foot pathology has been gathered, the following principles can guide the surgical correction plan.

1. Release or lengthen soft tissue to aid deformity correction
2. Prepare tendon transfers
3. Correct the hindfoot deformity
4. Correct the midfoot deformity if required
5. Correct the forefoot deformity if required
6. Secure tendon transfers at appropriate tension to correct residual deformity[6]

The rationale for this order is to first release the tight structures, including tendons, to facilitate correction, then to correct from proximal to distal, then to secure the tendon transfers at the end to balance the foot in its new position. It is also practically sensible to fix the tendon transfers at the end, where there is less manoeuvring of the foot, which can risk stretching or pulling out the transfer.

If we revisit the different cavus foot deformity patterns, management strategies can be broadly formulated bearing the above principles and deformity patterns in mind.

In rigid cavovarus feet with a hindfoot apex of deformity, either subtalar or triple arthrodesis is a reliable surgical option.[4] A subtalar fusion alone may be suitable in cases of milder hindfoot deformity but a triple fusion is a more reliable option in severe cases as the potential for deformity correction is greater.[4] Triple fusion in the cavovarus foot was first described by Ryerson in 1923.[11] A modification to the triple arthrodesis specifically for managing cavus feet was proposed by Siffert in 1966, called the beak triple arthrodesis.[12] Siffert's modification involved an osteotomy of the anterior calcaneus extending through the talar head and neck but retaining a shelf of bone at the dorsal talus. This shelf resembled a bird's beak, hence the name of the arthrodesis. The prepared navicular joint surface can then be positioned inferior to this beak and joint preparation can also take a dorsal closing wedge, accounting for correction of varus and supination.[4,12]

In the equinocavovarus foot, the management strategy is similar to the management of the cavovarus foot, however more attention must be paid to correction of the equinus deformity, which will limit progress if not addressed appropriately. This can be done by gastrocnemius recession or Achilles tendon lengthening procedures depending on which is tight as guided by the Silfverskiold test. If a plantigrade position of the ankle is not achievable after soft tissue release and lengthening, a good subsequent option is a Lambrinudi arthrodesis, where an anterior wedge is excised from the talus and calcaneus to permit hindfoot dorsiflexion and achievement of a plantigrade foot after subtalar fusion.[13] It is important to only correct the hindfoot to a neutral calcaneal pitch and not to over lengthen the Achilles to accommodate a concomitant midfoot cavus deformity (**Fig. 3**).

In pure cavus feet, correction only needs to be considered in the sagittal plane. If isolated plantar flexion of the first ray is causing the deformity, then one may opt for a dorsiflexion osteotomy to correct the pure cavus foot. But if the deformity is occurring at the talonavicular and calcaneocuboid joints or in the midfoot, then a Chopart or

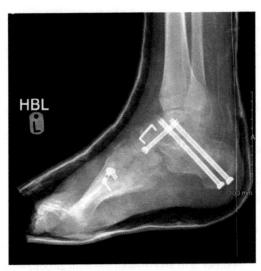

Fig. 3. Post-operative lateral radiograph illustrating a double hindfoot arthrodesis for a cavovarus foot deformity. Overcorrection of calcaneal pitch has been avoided., If the forefoot is excessively dorsiflexed, functional over lengthening of the Achilles tendon can occur.

midfoot arthrodesis at the apex of the deformity with a dorsal closing wedge may be a more suitable surgical option.[6]

When dealing with a calcaneocavus foot, the priority is refunctioning the Achilles tendon and overcoming weak hindfoot plantarflexion. This is a challenging task and can be done by transferring tibialis anterior to the Achilles tendon, but reported results are variable. The cavus portion of the deformity can be addressed similar to the suggestions above once Achilles function has been restored.[6]

For the remainder of this article, we will focus on managing the more common rigid cavovarus and equinocavovarus deformities, which will form the bulk of patients seen.

Our preferred technique for managing rigid hindfoot deformity in this cohort is to perform a double or triple arthrodesis. The calcaneocuboid joint is included if it has degenerative changes, or to aid in positioning of the lateral column if required.[3]

The patient is positioned supine with a thigh tourniquet and a sandbag under the ipsilateral buttock to raise the lateral hindfoot for surgical access. If the Achilles tendon is tight and the ankle cannot be brought to neutral, we perform a Hoke triple cut percutaneous Achilles tendon lengthening with two cuts medially and one cut laterally to minimise potential for sural nerve injury[14] (**Fig. 4**). If percutaneous Achilles lengthening will not suffice to achieve a plantigrade ankle, a formal open Achilles release can be performed via a posteromedial approach and Z-lengthening technique.[15] It is important the incision for the open Achilles lengthening is straight and does not curve distally, as a curve will lead to gapping of the wound after deformity correction, which can cause a difficult to manage soft tissue defect. We are also extremely cautious not to over lengthen the Achilles tendon, which can cause a calcaneus deformity.

Once the ankle can be brought to plantigrade, the sinus tarsi approach can be utilized to gain access to the subtalar joint. An incision is made from the base of the fibula in line with the 4th metatarsal. Subcutaneous dissection will reveal extensor digitorum brevis, which is elevated from its insertion to access the subtalar joint. The subtalar joint can now be prepared using flexible bone chisels. A laminar spreader can be

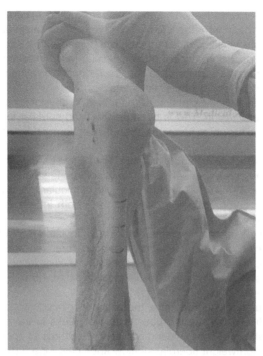

Fig. 4. Clinical photograph demonstrating skin incision markings for a Hoke triple-cut percutaneous Achilles tendon lengthening.

used to help to open up space in the subtalar joint to access the posterior, middle and anterior facets. Once the articular surfaces are fully denuded of cartilage and sclerotic subchondral bone to reveal cancellous bleeding bone, the surface is fenestrated using a 3.2 mm Kirschner wire and fish-scaled using a narrow osteotome. We in our institution term this process "petallising" the articular surface, as the end result of the prepared bony surface can look like the petals of a flower, increasing the available surface area for bony union.

After preparing the subtalar joint, the talonavicular joint is approached via our preference of a dorsal incision. Some authors propose a medial incision between tibialis anterior and tibialis posterior.[3,5] With our dorsal foot incision, extensor hallucis longus and tibialis anterior are palpated and marked on the skin and an incision is made between these landmarks. Sharp, deeper dissection between these two tendons is then performed, protecting them and in turn protecting the neurovascular bundle of dorsalis pedis and the deep peroneal nerve, which typically lies lateral to EHL at this level. The talonavicular joint capsule is divided to gain access to the joint and preparation of the articular surfaces is again performed in a systematic manner, with space being created between the surfaces using a laminar spreader or Hintermann retractor. The joint surfaces are denuded to subchondral bleeding bone and "petallised" as described above.

Finally, if the calcaneocuboid joint is identified as a potential pain generator, the lateral sinus tarsi incision is extended distally to adequately expose the calcaneocuboid joint and permit preparation after distraction using a Hintermann distractor. As is standard for our technique, the surfaces are "petallised" to promote joint surfaces favourable for arthrodesis.

The authors preferred reduction manoeuvre for a hindfoot fusion in a cavovarus foot is to push the talar head from the lateral side to reduce the talar head onto the navicular. Once the talonavicular joint is reduced, it is pinned with a Kirschner wire to hold the reduction. On occasion, once the talonavicular joint is reduced, a compression staple is applied from the lateral side to hold the reduction. We then proceed to formal fixation of the subtalar and talonavicular joints.

We usually fix the subtalar joint first, with the heel in physiological valgus, then proceed to talonavicular fusion. This is because the fixed subtalar joint will still allow a small degree of 'fine tuning' movements through the talonavicular joint, but the reverse is less possible.

Our preferred fixation of the subtalar joint is to use two partially threaded 8.0 mm or 6.5 mm cannulated screws, depending on available bone stock, passed from a stab incision in the heel. The screws should pass perpendicular to the prepared subtalar joint surfaces and compression is ideally seen in both intra-operative fluoroscopy and under direct vision in theatre.

The talonavicular joint can be stabilized using cannulated 5 mm partially threaded compression screws or a combination of partially threaded screws, compression plates and/or memory staples. The calcaneocuboid joint in our practice is most commonly stabilised and compressed using cannulated 4.5 mm partially threaded compression screws.

At the end of our surgical procedure, the patient is placed into a below knee backslab. Post-operatively, we see the patient at two weeks in the outpatient clinic to remove the backslab, check the wound and remove sutures as appropriate and place the patient into a lightweight fiberglass below knee cast for a further ten weeks. The patient is seen again in the clinic at the six-week post-surgery mark with the cast removed to assess the soft tissues and a new lightweight cast is applied at this stage. For the first four weeks post-surgery, we advise the patient is non-weight-bearing. For the middle four weeks, the patient can partially weight-bear in the cast and for the final four weeks, the patient can fully weight-bear through the cast. After twelve weeks, the patient is seen again in the outpatient clinic for radiographic assessment of deformity correction and assessment of bony union with a weight-bearing CT scan. Provided union and soft tissue healing is satisfactory, the patient will be provided with an Aircast boot and advised to fully weight-bear in the boot and wean out of the boot into their own comfortable and supportive footwear over the next 3 to 6 weeks. Based on the current evidence base for early weight bearing in hindfoot fusion, we are in the process of re-evaluating this regimen.

In some cases of more severe deformity, it may be necessary to excise wedges of bone when performing joint preparation in order to achieve a plantigrade foot with complete deformity correction. Given the varus nature of deformity, it is most common to take a lateral based wedge out of the calcaneocuboid joint, hence facilitating closing of the lateral column to correct any adductovarus deformity in the foot.[8] After this lateral wedge is excised, the calcaneocuboid joint fusion can be performed similar to the triple fusion fixation construct as suggested above.

ADJUNCTIVE PROCEDURES FOR SUCCESSFUL CAVUS CORRECTION

Whilst hindfoot arthrodesis techniques as outlined above are often important in the correction of the rigid cavovarus foot, it is essential to perform relevant adjunctive procedures alongside double or triple hindfoot arthrodesis to ensure success. Hindfoot arthrodesis alone is unlikely to work without balancing the deforming forces around the foot, as left unaddressed, there is a high chance of recurrent or persistent deformity.

It is firstly important to mention that in a rigid cavovarus foot where the apex of the deformity in the sagittal and/or axial plane is within the midfoot, a hindfoot fusion may not be indicated, and a midfoot wedge tarsectomy may be more appropriate. Similarly, there are a subset of cavovarus feet, where once the hindfoot is corrected, there remains midfoot adduction and rotation, and these may need combined hindfoot fusions with a wedge tarsectomy. It is the authors' experience that leaving a persistent midfoot adductus, despite hindfoot correction, may cause persistent pressure on the outer border of the foot and less satisfactory outcomes. Multiplanar corrections in the sagittal, axial and coronal plane via wedge tarsectomy can be complex, and a recent development in our practice is to use patient specific three-dimensional (3D) guided cutting jigs based on CT scans to plan the cuts to be as accurate as possible.[2,9,10] (**Fig. 5**). These can be particularly helpful where the computer planning can simulate the hindfoot correction and reveal the resultant midfoot deformity, to plan to extent of the tarsectomy and options for fixation.

There are multiple wedge tarsectomies described at different levels. Jahss described a dorsal wedge at the level of the tarsometatarsal joints and Cole and Japas both performed midfoot arthrodesis procedures after excising a dorsal wedge at the naviculocuneiform/cuboid level.[16–18] A dome osteotomy of the midfoot has also been described by Wilcox and Weiner, known as the Akron osteotomy, where again a wedge wider dorsally than plantarly is excised to correct the midfoot cavus deformity.[2,19] The specific techniques of these arthrodeses are beyond the scope of this hindfoot focused article.

Another set of essential adjunctive procedures that must be considered and performed where appropriate alongside hindfoot fusions for the cavovarus foot are tendon transfers and balancing. The most commonly transferred tendon is tibialis posterior.[4,20] In the CMT disease cavovarus foot, tibialis posterior and peroneus longus act excessively in relation to tibialis anterior and peroneus brevis, leading to an inversion and equinus force on the foot and ankle. If a hindfoot fusion procedure is done in isolation, there is a high chance of long-term failure of the procedure with recurrence of deformity owing to the persistent activity of tibialis posterior.[4,8,20]

In addition to a tibialis posterior tendon transfer, a peroneus longus to brevis tenodesis can also be a useful soft tissue balancing option alongside a tibialis posterior tendon transfer. Peroneus longus inserts on the plantar first metatarsal base and thus acts to plantarflex the first ray. In the cavovarus foot, the first ray is often plantarflexed, with a varus heel sometimes occurring secondary to this forefoot deformity (forefoot driven hindfoot varus). Alternatively, in a hindfoot driven pes cavus, plantarflexion of the first ray can occur to compensate for a rigid varus heel malalignment.[1] After correction of the hindfoot with an arthrodesis, the peroneus longus may continue to attempt to plantarflex the first ray and thus, removing this deforming force can be important to prevent future deformity recurrence, a principle we have now established.[8]

Our preferred technique for a tibialis posterior tendon transfer is via the interosseous route (**Fig. 6**). An incision is made centered on the navicular and the incision is extended proximally along the line of the tibialis posterior tendon. The tendon is identified within its sheath and the tendon sheath is split to expose the tendon. A tendon hook is used to isolate the tibialis posterior and the tendon is harvested as distal as possible from its navicular insertion. The tendon is then whip-stitched at its free end to create a neat distal tendon stump. A further medial incision is made approximately 5 cm proximal to the medial malleolus. The tibialis posterior tendon is identified in this level and again, the tendon is isolated within its sheath. The free whipstitched end of the tibialis posterior tendon is pulled out medially and delivered into this wound. The

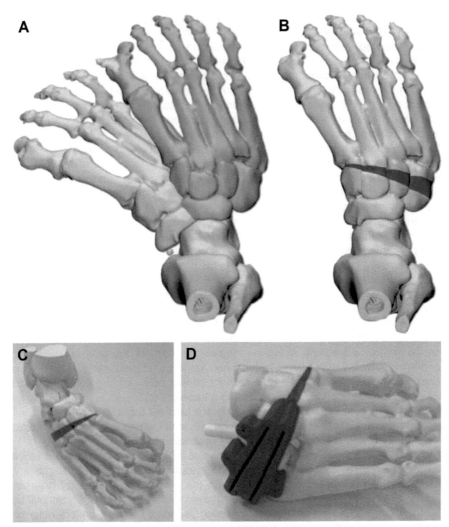

Fig. 5. Examples of wedge tarsectomy computer simulation based on three-dimensional CT planning, and a patient specific model and cutting guide produced from these computer simulations. (*A*) Computer simulation of forefoot position after hindfoot correction. (*B*) Computer simulation of midfoot wedge tarsectomy to achieve correction of residual forefoot adduction after hindfoot deformity correction. (*C*) Model based on computer simulation of midfoot wedge tarsectomy. (*D*) Model of midfoot wedge tarsectomy with patient specific cutting block in position to guide tarsectomy cut.

tendon is then routed between the tibia and fibula through the interosseous membrane, with a channel being made by passing curved Mayo scissors along the posterior border of the tibia. A corresponding incision is made laterally at the tip of the scissors and a tendon passer is used to deliver the tibialis posterior from the medial to lateral wound. Finally, the tibialis posterior tendon is routed to its distal insertion point. If tendon length is sufficient to permit insertion in the cuneiform bones distally, then the tendon end is sized and a tunnel is drilled in the appropriate cuneiform to

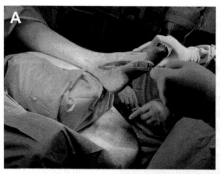
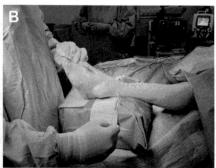
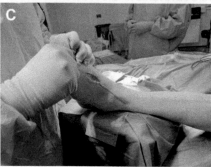

Fig. 6. Clinical photographs of tibialis posterior tendon transfer technique. (*A*) Medial approach and harvested, whip-stitched tibialis posterior tendon delivered into wound. (*B*) Tibialis posterior tendon transfer brought out through stab incision laterally after routing through interosseous membrane. (*C*) Length check of tibialis posterior tendon transfer with plan to fix tendon distally in cuneiform bone to balance foot position.

correspond to the width of the tibialis posterior tendon, with fixation with the appropriate size biotenodesis screw. We tend to use the lateral cuneiform to provide eversion and dorsiflexion, and the middle cuneiform if it is predominantly dorsiflexion required.

If the bone is osteopenic and may not accept a biotenodesis screw, or if the tendon does not have sufficient length to be inserted into the cuneiforms, then a tenodesis can be performed with the peroneus brevis tendon, to achieve the same goal of the converting the inverting varus pulling tibialis posterior to an everting tendon, thus balancing the forces around the fused hindfoot.

With reference to the peroneus longus, our technique is similar to that described by Myerson and colleagues, where peroneus longus is sutured to peroneus brevis at the distal fibula level. Once tenodesed, the longus is cut just distal to the tenodesis. The benefit of this technique is that it ensures the peroneus longus and brevis tendons remain at the appropriate tension before peroneus longus is cut.[8,20] An alternative is to cut the peroneus longus first and then suture its free proximal end to peroneus brevis at the same level. Both of these tenodesis procedures convert the action of peroneus longus from a plantarflexor of the first ray to an ankle everter, which exerts a favourable soft tissue balancing force in the setting of the corrected cavovarus foot deformity.[8]

A common additional procedure to permit cavovarus deformity correction is a plantar fascia release.[20] The rationale for a plantar fascia release is to free the calcaneus to permit correction of its varus position.[7] Myerson and colleagues suggest that it is helpful to perform a plantar fascia release first to overcome the rigidity caused by the contracted soft tissue. The suggestion in his article is to release the plantar fascia through a 1 cm incision adjacent to the heel, which can be accessed through the medial approach to the tibialis posterior tendon.[7] Whilst a plantar fascia release for managing the cavovarus foot is a well recognised procedure in the literature, our personal preference is to preserve the plantar fascia. In our experience, we have been able to achieve satisfactory deformity correction without sacrificing the stabilising function of the plantar fascia, which plays an important role in maintaining the plantar arch of the foot through the Windlass mechanism and enabling the foot to perform as a stable and rigid lever for forward propulsion in the gait cycle.[21]

After addressing severe cavovarus hindfoot deformities, there is often a pronation of the forefoot. This may be a prominent plantar flexed first ray. In such cases it is imperative to perform a forefoot balancing procedure such as a first metatarsal dorsiflexion osteotomy or first tarsometatarsal joint arthrodesis to restore the classic tripod of the foot between the first and fifth metatarsal heads and weight-bearing point of the os calcis[4] (**Fig. 7**).

It is also common for patients to have neurological imbalance of the toe extensors and flexors, leading to claw toes, which are characteristic in neurological conditions such as CMT. In such cases, flexor tenotomies in flexible deformities or corrective lesser toe fusions may be considered to prevent prominent areas of the toes rubbing plantarly or dorsally in footwear.[22] Similarly, plantarflexion at the hallux interphalangeal joint is also frequently seen in these patients and a Jones procedure can be

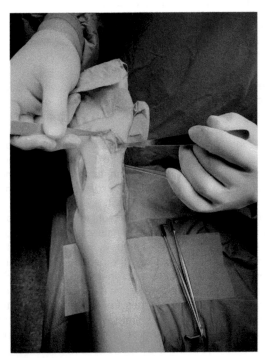

Fig. 7. First metatarsal basal dorsal closing wedge osteotomy to address plantar flexed first ray after hindfoot deformity correction.

undertaken, whereby the extensor hallucis longus is transferred to the neck of the first metatarsal, elevating the first ray. A later modification also added a hallux interphalangeal joint fusion, helping to correct the hallux clawing definitively.[22,23] It should be noted that forefoot procedures do not necessarily have to be undertaken at the time of hindfoot arthrodesis, due to the risks of causing excessive soft tissue swelling and wound issues, which can increase the risk of infection.[4]

SUMMARY

The key to a successful outcome of a hindfoot fusion is therefore multifaceted.

Firstly, a thorough clinical and radiographic assessment of the patient is essential prior to embarking on surgery. This is to achieve an understanding of the deformity and the deforming forces. This will ensure that the correct patients are selected for a hindfoot fusion in the setting of cavovarus and that the correct additional procedures are performed to enable a satisfactory and long-standing correction.

In this article, we have outlined several core principles of performing hindfoot arthrodesis in the cavovarus foot and outlined the authors preferred technique. We feel the key to success is to perform the correct additional procedures such as midfoot wedge tarsectomy, forefoot balancing and tendon transfers.

With this in mind, satisfying results can be achieved in this grateful patient cohort.

CLINICS CARE POINTS

- Thorough assessment of osseous deformity, degeneration and tendon balance is essential.
- Plan correction from proximal to distal.
- Consider apex of deformity in antero-posterior and sagittal plane.

REFERENCES

1. Maynou C, Szymanski C, Thiounn A. The adult cavus foot. EFORT Open Rev 2017;2(5):221–9.
2. Qin B, Wu S, Zhang H. Evaluation and management of cavus foot in adults: a narrative review. J Clin Med 2022;11(13). https://doi.org/10.3390/JCM11133679.
3. Mortenson KE, Fallat LM. Principles of triple arthrodesis and limited arthrodesis in the cavus foot. Clin Podiatr Med Surg 2021;38(3):411–25.
4. Kaplan JRM, Aiyer A, Cerrato RA, et al. Operative treatment of the cavovarus foot. Foot Ankle Int 2018;39(11):1370–82.
5. Zide JR, Myerson MS. Arthrodesis for the cavus foot. When, where, and how? Foot Ankle Clin 2013;18(4):755–67.
6. Wenz W. Double and triple tarsal fusions in the complex cavovarus foot. Foot Ankle Clin 2022;27(4):819–33.
7. Myerson MS, Myerson CL. Managing the complex cavus foot deformity. Foot Ankle Clin 2020;25(2):305–17.
8. Li S, Myerson MS. Failure of surgical treatment in patients with cavovarus deformity: why does this happen and how do we approach treatment? Foot Ankle Clin 2019;24(2):361–70.
9. Dagneaux L, Canovas F. 3D printed patient-specific cutting guide for anterior midfoot tarsectomy. Foot Ankle Int 2020;41(2):211–5.

10. Sobrón FB, Dos Santos-Vaquinhas A, Alonso B, et al. Technique tip: 3D printing surgical guide for pes cavus midfoot osteotomy. Foot Ankle Surg 2022;28(3): 371–7.

11. Ryerson EW. Arthrodesing operations on the feet : Edwin W. Ryerson MD (1872-1961). The 1st President of the AAOS 1932. Clin Orthop Relat Res 2008; 466(1):5–14.

12. Siffert R, Forster RI, Nachamie B. "Beak" triple arthrodesis for correction of severe cavus deformity. Clin Orthop Relat Res 1966;45:101–6.

13. So LWN, Kuong EE, To KTM, et al. Long-term outcome after Lambrinudi arthrodesis: how they're doing after three decades. J Orthop Surg 2019;27(1):1–7.

14. Hatt RN, Lamphier TA. Triple hemisection: a simplified procedure for lengthening the achilles tendon. N Engl J Med 1947;236(5):166–9.

15. Chen L, Greisberg J. Achilles lengthening procedures. Foot Ankle Clin 2009; 14(4):627–37.

16. Jahss MH. Tarsometatarsal truncated-wedge arthrodesis for pes cavus and equinovarus deformity of the fore part of the foot. J Bone Joint Surg Am 1980;62(5): 713–22.

17. Cole WH. The treatment of claw-foot. J Bone Joint Surg Am 1940;22(4):3–6.

18. Japas LM. Surgical treatment of pes cavus by tarsal V-osteotomy: preliminary report. J Bone Joint Surg Am 1968;50(5):927–44.

19. Wilcox PG, Weiner DS. The Akron midtarsal dome osteotomy in the treatment of rigid pes cavus: a preliminary review. J Pediatr Orthop 1985;5(3):333–8.

20. Myerson MS, Myerson CL. Cavus foot: deciding between osteotomy and arthrodesis. Foot Ankle Clin 2019;24(2):347–60.

21. Malhotra K, Davda K, Singh D. The pathology and management of lesser toe deformities. EFORT Open Rev 2016;1(11):409–19.

22. Nogueira MP, Farcetta F, Zuccon A. Cavus foot. Foot Ankle Clin 2015;20(4): 645–56.

23. Jones R III. The soldier's foot and the treatment of comon deformities of the foot. Br Med J 1916;1(2891):749–53.

Tibiotalocalcaneal and Tibiotalar Arthrodesis for Severe Cavovarus Deformity
Tips and Tricks

Inês Casais, MD[a], Anny Steenwerckx, MD[b], Kristian Buedts, MD[c,d,*]

KEYWORDS

- Cavovarus foot • Varus ankle • Ankle arthrodesis • Tibiotalar arthrodesis
- Tibiotalocalcaneal arthrodesis

KEY POINTS

- Varus ankle arthritis is the most common, whether resulting from cavovarus foot or other causes. Associated midfoot and forefoot deformities must be considered for a successful treatment.
- A thorough clinical history and physical examination is important, and the main steps are described in this article.
- Weight-bearing computed tomography is valuable for preoperative planning, 3-dimensional analysis and creation of patient-specific instrumentation.
- Tibiotalocalcaneal arthrodesis may be preferrable to isolated tibiotalar fusion.
- The authors present a curved anterolateral incision for tibiotalocalcaneal arthrodesis and a method of partial fibula bridging onlay grafting.

 Video content accompanies this article at http://www.foot.theclinics.com.

INTRODUCTION

Varus ankle deformity may progress from cavovarus foot or may originate from the ankle itself, mostly in posttraumatic cases, including fractures and ligament lesions. However, it is interesting to notice that, even in primary and secondary atraumatic ankle arthritis, varus alignment predominates.[1]

a Serviço de Ortopedia, Orthopedics and Traumatology Department, Centro Hospitalar de Vila Nova de Gaia e Espinho, Rua Conceição Fernandes, Vila Nova de Gaia 4434-502, Portugal; b Orthopaedics and Traumatology Department, AZ Diest, Statiestraat 65, Diest 3290, Belgium; c Foot and Ankle Unit, Orthopedics and Traumatology Department, ZNA Middelheim, Antwerpen, Belgium; d Gewrichtskliniek, Jos Ratinckxstraat 1 bus 53, 2600 Berchem, Belgium
* Corresponding author. Gewrichtskliniek, Jos Ratinckxstraat 1 bus 53, 2600 Berchem, Belgium
E-mail address: k.buedts@telenet.be

Foot Ankle Clin N Am 28 (2023) 819–831
https://doi.org/10.1016/j.fcl.2023.06.003
1083-7515/23/© 2023 Elsevier Inc. All rights reserved.

In cases of rigid deformities and debilitating osteoarthritis where conservative treatment has failed, joint-sparing realignment procedures have no place. In these complex cases, arthrodesis is the best choice, as it allows for deformity correction with reliable pain relief.[2] There are various surgical techniques and associated procedures that can be used, and several factors, including deformity and patient specific considerations, should be taken into account to achieve the best possible result.

This article provides a systematic approach to the varus ankle, focusing on treatment strategies for the most severe cases through arthrodesis and providing useful tips and tricks.

CAUSE

The most common causes for varus ankle arthritis can be classified as muscle imbalance, ligament insufficiency, bone deformity, or a combination of these factors.[3]

Starting with muscle imbalance, a forefoot-driven cavovarus foot often results from neurological conditions (such as seen in upper and lower motor neuron diseases) but may also be idiopathic. A muscle imbalance between the peroneal muscle group and the tibialis posterior causes a shift of the first ray into plantar flexion and the hindfoot into varus. The Achilles tendon vector will secondarily aggravate the hindfoot's medial deviation, and associated ankle equinus may develop due to shortening of the gastrocnemius. These changes lead to abnormal weight distribution in the ankle joint and predominantly medial degenerative changes.[4]

Trauma, however, is the most common cause for varus ankle arthritis.[1] It can affect the ligaments, resulting in chronic lateral ankle instability, or the bones, particularly in cases of malleolar and tibial pilon fractures. In cases of ligament insufficiency, the deformity is driven by the hindfoot, and the forefoot typically compensates by pronation through peroneus longus overaction and first ray plantar flexion. In cases of fractures, malunion leads to varus malalignment of the affected bones.[3]

Primary and secondary atraumatic ankle arthritis also demonstrate a predominantly varus alignment.[1]

In addition, proximal limb deformities, especially tibial shaft fractures, may also cause varus deviation of the distal segment.[3]

ASSESSMENT AND PLANNING

Table 1 provides a summary of essential points in the assessment and planning of treatment of severe cavovarus deformity.

Table 1 Clinics care points—assessment and planning in severe cavovarus deformity	
Clinical History	Previous surgeries Previous trauma Neurological disease
Physical Examination	Soft tissue problems Coleman block test Midfoot and forefoot passive mobility Passive ankle dorsiflexion and Silfverskiöld test Search for peroneal tendon pain
Preoperative Studies	Weightbearing CT scan; possibly patient-specific instrumentation MRI to search for cartilage damage, bone edema, or tendon lesions Vascular evaluation Laboratory studies (comorbidity control)

Clinical History and Physical Examination

A comprehensive patient history can contribute to identifying the cause of the deformity. It is important to investigate the family history of neurological diseases and the personal history of trauma. Being aware of associated comorbidities such as diabetes, vascular disease, and smoking can influence surgical decision-making and help anticipate and prevent possible complications.[5] It is crucial to advise smokers to quit smoking due to the higher risk of wound problems and nonunion associated with smoking.[6]

A thorough physical examination is essential and should include the following:

- Observation of shoe wear pattern: this can help identify abnormal weight distribution, with excessive lateral wear of the heel of the shoes being common in varus alignment.[5]
- Standing posture examination: evaluating the patient from the front, side and back allows 3-dimensional classification of the ankle, hindfoot, midfoot, and forefoot position. Common findings include prominence of the lateral malleolus, the "Peek-a-boo" heel sign, and a high foot arch. The Coleman block test is important for differentiating correctable from fixed hindfoot varus and is crucial for determining the appropriate treatment.[7] If possible, assessing the patient during single-leg stance can be helpful, as it avoids compensation from the contralateral limb. Podoscopy, if available, is a useful tool.
- Gait and active muscular strength examination (Video 1): observing the patient during gait can reveal subtle changes in muscle strength. Muscle strength should be assessed using the Medical Research Council Manual Muscle Test.[7]
- Passive mobility range of the various lower limb joints: assessing subtalar flexibility is important due to its therapeutic implications. The correctability of midfoot and forefoot deformities should be evaluated to determine the need for additional osteotomies. Ankle equinus is commonly present, and the Silfverskiöld test is used to identify isolated gastrocnemius contracture, which should be properly addressed.[5]
- Palpation and provocative maneuvers: digital palpation can identify painful points not only in the affected joints but also in surrounding soft tissue, providing clues to common associated problems such as fifth metatarsal stress fractures, plantar fasciitis, Achilles tendinopathy, and peroneal tendinopathy. Provocative maneuvers can identify additional problems including ankle or subtalar instability and peroneal tendon subluxation.[7]
- Skin and soft tissue examination: callus formation indicates excessive pressure, and its location is an important clue to its cause. Arterial and venous disease stigmata should be sought, in anticipation of surgical complications. The presence of scars may indicate previous surgeries and has implications for future incision planning.

Preoperative Workup

When it comes to imaging studies, the following should be considered.

- Standard radiographs: these should include a full-length weight-bearing lower limb radiograph; standing dorsoplantar and lateral views of the foot; and standing posteroanterior, lateral, and Meary or Saltzman views of the ankle.
- A standardized frontal full-leg view with the patella facing forward is necessary to evaluate the lower leg mechanical axis and to appreciate any other deformity or surgery in the lower limb.

- Weight-bearing computed tomography (WBCT): this imaging modality allows for a comprehensive 3-dimensional assessment of the deformity and evaluation of the articular surfaces[8,9] (**Fig. 1**).
- MRI: it is valuable for evaluating articular damage in adjacent joints, which may be underestimated with CT. It is also useful for identifying soft tissue lesions, particularly in the lateral ligaments and peroneal tendons.[10] MRI provides detailed information on soft tissue structures.

By using these imaging modalities, clinicians can obtain a comprehensive evaluation of the deformity, assess the condition of articular surfaces, and detect any associated soft tissue abnormalities.

Laboratory studies should be conducted to assess the control of comorbidities in patients; this may include checking for anemia or platelet abnormalities through a hemogram, evaluating diabetes control with hemoglobin A1C levels, and assessing for active infection using C-reactive protein and erythrocyte sedimentation rate. It is important to assess the nutritional status of the patient, including the levels of vitamin D.[11]

A vascular assessment should be undertaken through Doppler ultrasonography or angio-CT.[12]

Indications for Arthrodesis

Severe cavovarus foot is a disabling condition for the patient. Often conservative treatment with bracing and orthopaedic footwear fails to provide good functionality for patients due to the unbraceble 3-dimensional deformity present in the foot and ankle segment.

The surgical treatment aims to achieve a painless, plantigrade foot that allows weight-bearing and functional gait while wearing shoes.

For flexible varus ankles, joint-sparing procedures can be performed. These procedures involve soft tissue releases and tendon transfers to balance the forces acting on the joints and realignment osteotomies to adjust the weight-bearing axes.[13]

In selected patients with correctable deformities, appropriate age (>50 years), functional status, and adequate soft tissue conditions and bone stock, ankle arthroplasty may be considered. In some cases, arthroplasty can be combined with osteotomies and/or ligament repair to achieve a well-aligned and stable joint.[14,15]

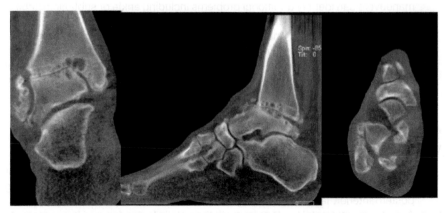

Fig. 1. The WBCT scan reveals a degenerative and painful cavovarus deformity characterized by significant degeneration and anteromedial rotation of the talus, causing it to deviate outside the tibiotalar joint.

Arthrodesis is indicated when conservative treatment has been ineffective, and there are adequate soft tissue conditions, sufficient bone stock, and no active infection or medical comorbidities that would contraindicate surgery.

Preoperative Planning

WBCT is extensively used in preoperative planning. It serves as a valuable diagnostic tool, allowing imaging of the foot and ankle under more physiological weight-bearing conditions. WBCT provides information on the position of the talus in the ankle mortise while the patient is bearing weight. This enables visualization of various bony impingements and clear spaces within the ankle joints. In addition, in combination with distance mapping techniques (**Fig. 2**), WBCT can reveal rotational deformities of the talus and coxa pedis (including the talonavicular joints and subtalar joints). It allows for the calculation of different axes. Importantly, WBCT also shows the position of the foot in relation to the coxa pedis and ankle under load.

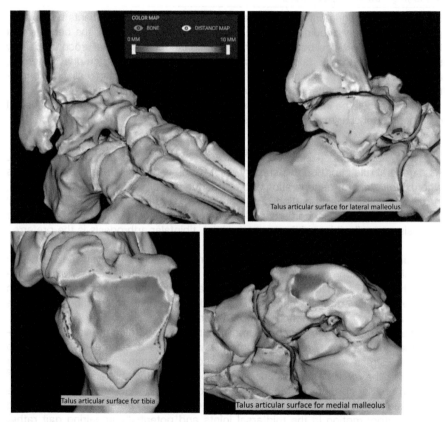

Fig. 2. After generating the WBCT images, a 3-dimensional model of the cavovarus foot deformity can be constructed. The model displays the lateral traction osteophytes. The color scale on the model represents the distance mapping between the talus and tibia in the tibiotalar joint. It clearly demonstrates the rotation of the talus out of its normal articulation. These osteophytes need to be removed, along with a medial release, in order to facilitate the reduction of the talus back into the ankle mortise.

The use of volume rendering software facilitates the creation of digital 3-dimensional prints, which can be immensely helpful in preoperative planning. These prints aid in visualizing the anatomy and understanding the deformity.[16]

In certain cases, patient-specific cutting guides can be created using WBCT; this is particularly useful when a corrective tarsectomy is planned for a rigid cavus foot and when an elevation osteotomu of the first ray metatarsal osteotomy alone cannot adequately address the deformity.[17,18]

The authors use a combination of WBCT scan and a standard MRI protocol in their evaluations. This approach allows a comprehensive assessment of the soft tissue envelope, ligamentous integrity, and identification of any tendon pathologies. Furthermore, it provides valuable information on the quality of the cartilage and helps detect the presence of any bony edema, which provides biological insight into the condition. The combination of WBCT and MRI enables a more thorough evaluation of both the bony and soft tissue structures, contributing to a comprehensive understanding of the patient's condition.

Managing Patient Expectations

Expectation management is considered of utmost importance. Patients undergoing joint fusion surgery should have a clear understanding not only of the benefits that the surgery will provide but also of the limitations inherent to the procedure. They should be aware that certain activities, such as kneeling, walking on uneven terrain, and descending stairs, may present difficulties after surgery. Setting realistic expectations helps patients better navigate the postsurgical period.

Patients should be informed that despite undergoing corrective surgery, the use of orthopedic footwear may still be necessary.

How to Decide Between Tibiotalar and Tibiotalocalcaneal Arthrodesis

As a general rule in orthopedic surgery, joint fusion is typically reserved for patients who exhibit signs of degeneration and corresponding clinical symptoms. Therefore, in cases involving degeneration of the ankle and subtalar joints, tibiotalocalcaneal (TTC) arthrodesis is the recommended procedure. For patients with isolated tibiotalar arthrosis and a flexible, painless subtalar joint, tibiotalar arthrodesis is the preferred choice.

Evaluation of the subtalar joint should be conducted through physical examination (assessing inversion/eversion movements with the ankle joint at a 90° angle) and imaging studies (CT scan to observe joint space narrowing, osteophytes, and sclerosis in cases of subtalar arthritis, whereas MRI provides better characterization of cartilage lesions and may reveal subchondral bone edema).

However, there has been debate among surgeons regarding the value of preserving the subtalar joint, as it can potentially become a source of pain due to increased stress following ankle fusion (secondary degeneration of the subtalar joint being the most common cause for reoperation after tibiotalar arthrodesis).[19] Furthermore, according to Monteagudo and colleagues,[20] after isolated ankle fusion, the action of the triceps surae muscle can lead to subtalar varus, restricting compensatory motion in the midtarsal joints and potentially impairing gait rather than improving it.

Considering these factors, the authors believe that in most cases of severe varus ankle arthritis, patients will benefit more from TTC arthrodesis, which allows control of the subtalar position, facilitates midfoot motion, and potentially reduces the need for future revision surgeries.

Additional Procedures

As discussed in the "Cause" section, varus ankle deformity often coexists with other foot and ankle deformities. The goal of the surgery is to achieve a plantigrade foot that is well aligned, stable, and free of pain.

In cases where there are advanced degenerative changes in adjacent joints, especially the talonavicular joint, a pantalar arthrodesis may be necessary.[21]

For addressing cavus deformity, a plantar fascia release performed through a mini-medial approach can be beneficial. In situations involving fixed forefoot malalignment, various osteotomies can be used. The typical deformities include cavus, forefoot pronation, and forefoot adduction. It is crucial to identify the apex of the deformity through weight-bearing imaging studies, as performing the osteotomy at this specific point yields better outcomes. A dorsal closing wedge osteotomy of the first ray (first metatarsal or medial cuneiform) can correct both cavus and pronation, provided that the Chopart joint is flexible. In more rigid cases, a larger multiplanar tarsal osteotomy, such as the Japas osteotomy, may be required.[22] Planning these corrective osteotomies can be complex, and the authors have used patient-specific instrumentation to achieve predictable results (**Fig. 3**).

If an equinus deformity is present and is not amenable to correction through preoperative physical therapy, Achilles lengthening should be performed to achieve neutral dorsiflexion of the ankle.[4]

THE AUTHORS' PREFERRED SURGICAL TECHNIQUE

There are various surgical approaches and fixation methods available for arthrodesis in varus ankles. In this article, a brief overview of the available options is provided, and a preferred method is recommended by the authors. **Table 2** provides a summary of the authors' tips and tricks for surgical treatment of severe cavovarus deformity.

Approach

The surgical approach in patients with varus ankles can be challenging due to various factors such as soft tissue retraction, chronic ulcers, previous scars, implants, and increased risk of wound complications in certain patient populations. Different approaches including lateral transfibular, anterior, medial, posterior, and posterolateral approaches have been described.[23] Although arthroscopic joint preparation is possible, it may not be suitable for significant deformities.[24] According to the authors, the choice of approach is important not only for accessing the joint surfaces but also

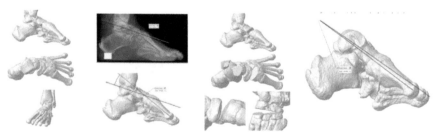

Fig. 3. The 3D images generated from the WBCT scan illustrate the presence of cavus deformity in the midfoot, characterized by supination and adduction. A virtual osteotomy was performed to address this deformity. A biplanar osteotomy, combining a medial and dorsal closing wedge effect, is implemented to effectively reduce the deformity. The osteotomy is realized with patient-specific instrumentation (PSI) guides.

Table 2
Clinics care points—authors' tips and tricks for treatment of severe cavovarus deformity

Type of Arthrodesis	TTC fusion is the preferred method in most cases: good deformity correction, avoids reoperation for future subtalar fusion, allows optimal subtalar positioning for the best postoperative midfoot mobility
Surgical Approach and Technique	Anterolateral curved approach allows full visualization and preparation of subtalar and ankle joint, fibular osteotomy, and reduces skin problems
	Gutter and soft tissue release is essential to correct the deformities while sparing bone
	Do not forget the foot deformity: talonavicular joint, cavus, adduction and pronation should be assessed and addressed
	Achilles and plantar fascia elongation may be needed
Implants and Grafting	Anterior plate and screws for improved stability
	Locked fixation for osteoporotic bone
	A partial fibula graft is preferred by the authors
	Consider augmentation with demineralized bone matrix powder and iliac crest bone marrow aspirate
	In large defects, iliac crest autograft or allograft may be needed

for facilitating adequate soft tissue release and debridement, which aids in bone-sparing deformity correction.

In cases of isolated tibiotalar fusion, the authors prefer a direct anterior approach to the ankle, allowing thorough preparation of the articular surfaces and avoiding previous osteosynthesis incisions that are often present.

However, for TTC arthrodesis, the senior author has developed an alternative incision (**Fig. 4**) that provides wide access to the anterior and lateral ankle, with good access to the medial ankle, subtalar joint, and midfoot.

The incision starts approximately 15 cm proximal to the tip of the fibula, anterior to the fibula, and curves posteriorly from the fibula. At the fibula point, it follows a line from the distal end of the fibula to the base of the sinus tarsi, extending toward the base of the fourth metatarsal. The deep proximal dissection is performed between the extensor digitorum longus and the peroneus brevis muscles. The inferior extensor retinaculum is divided near the fibula, whereas the superficial peroneal nerve remains in the anterior

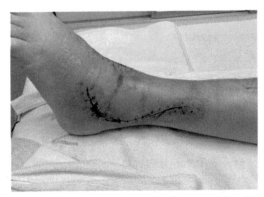

Fig. 4. The wound 2 weeks after the initial surgery. The curved-lined incision and an additional anteromedial incision can be observed.

flap. The fibula is then completely exposed, and the deep dissection in the distal part occurs between the superficial peroneal nerve and the sural nerve. At the level of the syndesmosis, an anterior flap is raised to expose the anterior tibiotalar joint.

If it is planned to osteotomize the fibula, this is performed at this stage. The syndesmosis and anterior talofibular and calcaneofibular ligaments are taken down, whereas the sural nerve and saphenous vein are left in the posterior flap part of the wound. This provides broad access to the tibiotalar and subtalar joints.

In cases where the access to the medial gutter is insufficient through the primary surgical approach, an additional medial incision can be made specifically over the medial gutter. This additional incision allows for better visualization and access to the medial aspect of the ankle and the talonavicular joint, facilitating adequate debridement and correction of deformities.

It is crucial that the surgical incisions provide sufficient access to the lateral, anterior, and medial aspects of the ankle joint, which allows for effective release and debridement of the affected area, removal of osteophytes, and performance of necessary soft tissue releases. By ensuring adequate exposure, the surgeon can properly reduce the talus within the ankle mortise.

Implants

A wide range of implants can be used for joint fusion procedures, including screws, staples, plates, intramedullary nails, and external fixators. The selection of the implant depends on various factors such as the surgical approach, soft tissue condition, and the surgeon's expertise. Several research studies have tried to demonstrate superiority of one method compared with others.[25–27] However, there is a lack of high-quality clinical evidence, and it is challenging to make direct comparisons due to the significant variation in surgical techniques used.[28]

The authors' preferred implant choice is an anterior low-profile plate (**Fig. 5**), which offers compression of the articular surfaces and additional locked screws. This implant configuration provides enhanced stability, particularly in cases where the bone is osteoporotic.

Use of Graft

The authors' preferred technique involves a high fibular osteotomy. Subsequently, the fibula is divided into 2 parts, with the medial part being used as an autograft and the lateral part being preserved (**Fig. 6**). Cancellous bone graft is collected from the resected segment, and the remaining corticocancellous part is used as an onlay graft, which is fixed to the tibia and talus using compression screws (see **Fig. 5**). This approach allows for deformity correction, graft collection, and potentially promotes fusion through a larger area of bone contact. It also preserves stability, reducing the risk of valgus failure, and minimizes the risk of damage to the peroneal tendons. In cases with significant bone defects, autograft harvested from the iliac crest or allograft can be added as needed.

In addition, the authors use biological enhancement of fusion by using demineralized bone matrix powder along with bone marrow aspirate from the ipsilateral iliac crest. This approach aims to optimize the fusion process and potentially improve outcomes.

Postoperative Protocol

Postoperative antibiotic prophylaxis is administered for a duration of 24 hours to prevent infection. Following surgery, the patients are placed in a backslab splint for a period of 2 weeks. At the end of this period, the dressing is removed, and the wounds

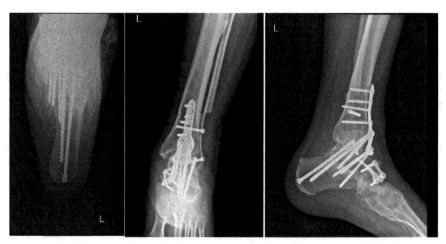

Fig. 5. A TTC fusion is depicted, following the authors' preferred method. The joint is accessed through the anterolateral incision, and an anterior stabilization plate is used. The lateral portion of the fibula is used as a bridging autograft, secured with compression screws to the proximal tibia and distal talus. Furthermore, an additional tarsectomy was performed to address the cavus foot, using patient-specific cutting guides and stabilization with a medial plate, conducted through the medial incision.

are assessed. If there are no signs of wound complications or infection, the patient is transitioned to a closed non–weight-bearing cast in a neutral position for an additional 2 weeks.

After a total of 4 weeks postsurgery, the patient's treatment plan involves transferring to a walking cast, allowing for gradual weight-bearing as tolerated by the patient. This walking cast is worn for an additional 4 weeks. Throughout this phase, the patient is encouraged to bear weight on the affected foot as much as they can comfortably tolerate.

As part of the follow-up process, bony union progress is monitored through radiographs. In addition, at around 6 months postoperative, a WBCT scan is performed to confirm the establishment of bony union.

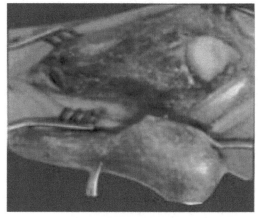

Fig. 6. Preoperative picture of the high fibula osteotomy and the divided fibula, where the posteriorly fixed lateral part will serve as an autograft bridging plate.

Physical therapy plays a crucial role in the postoperative rehabilitation process. In the absence of midfoot arthrodesis, the focus of physical therapy should be on improving flexibility in the forefoot and midfoot.

Physical therapy also includes training the patient to walk with an ankle fusions, as this is an important aspect of restoring functional gait. The therapy sessions may involve gait training exercises and techniques to help the patient adapt to the changes in their foot and ankle mechanics.

In addition to the therapeutic exercises, antiedema therapy may be initiated to manage any swelling that may occur after surgery. This therapy may include techniques such as elevation, compression therapy, and manual lymphatic drainage to reduce edema and promote optimal healing.

SUMMARY

Varus ankle deformity can arise in various circumstances, and when it leads to arthritis, surgical intervention may be necessary. Before surgery, patients should undergo a thorough evaluation, taking into account the underlying cause and associated issues. It is crucial to assess vascular health and effectively manage any comorbidities. In complex cases, arthrodesis often provides a viable solution, and TTC fusion is the preferred approach for the authors, as it minimizes complications related to the subtalar joint.

Surgeons must ensure that patients have realistic expectations regarding the outcomes of these surgical procedures. When planning for surgery, WBCT images should be used for a comprehensive assessment, considering not only the ankle but also midfoot and forefoot deformities. Patient-specific instrumentation can be beneficial in optimizing surgical planning and execution. The authors introduce a curved anterolateral incision technique, which allows for thorough debridement of both the ankle and subtalar joint, facilitates the placement of an anterior plate, and potentially reduces the risk of skin complications associated with dual incisions. Partial fibula bridging onlay grafting is used to aid in deformity correction, enhance stability, and prevent damage to the peroneal tendons.

Although managing varus ankle deformities can be complex, the authors hold the belief that with systematic evaluation, meticulous planning, and comprehensive surgical procedures, favorable outcomes can be achieved.

CONFLICT OF INTEREST

The authors have nothing to disclose.

SUPPLEMENTARY DATA

Supplementary data related to this article can be found online at https://doi.org/10.1016/j.fcl.2023.06.003.

REFERENCES

1. Valderrabano V, Horisberger M, Russell I, et al. Etiology of ankle osteoarthritis. Clin Orthop Relat Res 2009;467(7):1800–6.
2. Ewalefo SO, Dombrowski M, Hirase T, et al. Management of posttraumatic ankle arthritis: literature review. Current Reviews in Musculoskeletal Medicine 2018; 11(4):546–57.
3. AlSayel F, Valderrabano V. Arthrodesis of a varus ankle. Foot Ankle Clin 2019; 24(2):265–80.

4. DiDomenico LA, Abdelfattah S, Chan D, et al. The cavovarus ankle: approaches to ankle instability and inframalleolar deformity. Clin Podiatr Med Surg 2021;38(3): 461–81.

5. Maynou C, Szymanski C, Thiounn A. The adult cavus foot. EFORT Open Reviews 2017;2(5):221–9.

6. Heyes G, Weigelt L, Molloy A, et al. The influence of smoking on foot and ankle surgery: a review of the literature. Foot 2021;46:101735.

7. Akoh CC, Phisitkul P. Clinical examination and radiographic assessment of the cavus foot. Foot Ankle Clin 2019;24(2):183–93.

8. Barg A, Bailey T, Richter M, et al. Weightbearing computed tomography of the foot and ankle: emerging technology topical review. Foot Ankle Int 2018;39(3): 376–86.

9. Bernasconi A, Cooper L, Lyle S, et al. Intraobserver and interobserver reliability of cone beam weightbearing semi-automatic three-dimensional measurements in symptomatic pes cavovarus. Foot Ankle Surg 2020;26(5):564–72.

10. Park HJ, Cha SD, Kim HS, et al. Reliability of MRI findings of peroneal tendinopathy in patients with lateral chronic ankle instability. Clin Orthop Surg 2010;2(4): 237–43.

11. Ramanathan D, Berkowitz MJ, Davis A, et al. Vitamin D deficiency and outcomes after ankle fusion. Foot Ankle Orthop 2020;5(4).

12. Conti MS, Savenkov O, Ellis SJ. Association of peripheral vascular disease with complications after total ankle arthroplasty. Foot Ankle Orthop 2019;4(2). https://doi.org/10.1177/2473011419843379. 2473011419843379.

13. Barton T, Winson I. Joint sparing correction of cavovarus feet in charcot-marie-tooth disease: what are the limits? Foot Ankle Clin 2013;18(4):673–88.

14. Trajkovski T, Pinsker E, Cadden A, et al. Outcomes of ankle arthroplasty with pre-operative coronal-plane varus deformity of 10° or greater. J Bone Joint Surg Am 2013;95(15):1382–8.

15. Shock RP, Christensen JC, Schuberth JM. Total ankle replacement in the varus ankle. J Foot Ankle Surg 2011;50(1):5–10.

16. Kadakia RJ, Wixted CM, Allen NB, et al. Clinical applications of custom 3D printed implants in complex lower extremity reconstruction. 3D Printing in Medicine 2020;6(1):29.

17. Sobrón FB, Dos Santos-Vaquinhas A, Alonso B, et al. Technique tip: 3D printing surgical guide for pes cavus midfoot osteotomy. Foot Ankle Surg 2022;28(3): 371–7.

18. Dagneaux L, Canovas F. 3D printed patient-specific cutting guide for anterior midfoot tarsectomy. Foot Ankle Int 2020;41(2):211–5.

19. Ling JS, Smyth NA, Fraser EJ, et al. Investigating the relationship between ankle arthrodesis and adjacent-joint arthritis in the hindfoot: a systematic review. J Bone Joint Surg Am 2015;97(6):513–20.

20. Monteagudo M, Martínez-de-Albornoz P. Deciding between ankle and tibiotalo-calcaneal arthrodesis for isolated Ankle. Arthritis. Foot and Ankle Clinics 2022; 27(1):217–31.

21. Chawla S, Brage M. Pantalar arthrodesis. Foot Ankle Clin 2022;27(4):883–95.

22. Nogueira MP, Farcetta F, Zuccon A. Cavus foot. Foot Ankle Clin 2015;20(4): 645–56.

23. Martínez-de-Albornoz P, Monteagudo M. Tibiotalocalcaneal arthrodesis in severe hindfoot deformities. Foot Ankle Clin 2022/12/01/2022;27(4):847–66.

24. Leucht A-K, Veljkovic A. Arthroscopic ankle arthrodesis. Foot Ankle Clin 2022; 27(1):175–97.

25. Hamid KS, Glisson RR, Morash JG, et al. Simultaneous intraoperative measurement of cadaver ankle and subtalar joint compression during arthrodesis with intramedullary nail, screws, and tibiotalocalcaneal plate. Foot Ankle Int 2018;39(9): 1128–32.

26. Chiodo CP, Acevedo JI, Sammarco VJ, et al. Intramedullary rod fixation compared with blade-plate-and-screw fixation for tibiotalocalcaneal arthrodesis: a biomechanical investigation. J Bone Joint Surg Am 2003;85(12):2425–8.

27. Lee AT, Sundberg EB, Lindsey DP, et al. Biomechanical comparison of blade plate and intramedullary nail fixation for tibiocalcaneal arthrodesis. Foot Ankle Int 2010;31(2):164–71.

28. van den Heuvel SBM, Doorgakant A, Birnie MFN, et al. Open ankle arthrodesis: a systematic review of approaches and fixation methods. Foot Ankle Surg 2021; 27(3):339–47.

Total Ankle Replacement in Cavovarus Deformity
How Far Can We Go?

Jean M. Brilhault, MD, PhD[a],*, Gaspard Auboyneau, MD[b],
Louis Rony, MD, PhD[c]

KEYWORDS

- Cavovarus • Varus deformity • Total ankle replacement • Total ankle arthroplasty

KEY POINTS

- Despite cavovarus preoperative deformity, satisfactory results can be obtained with total ankle replacement (TAR) if alignment and balance are obtained.
- Correction of varus malalignment may be performed at the time of TAR or as a 2-stage procedure.
- Ancillary procedures are key to successful functional results and satisfactory implant survival for TAR in cases with cavovarus deformity.

INTRODUCTION

Because of the good functional results and satisfactory implant survival achieved with modern models, total ankle replacement (TAR) has become a legitimate alternative to ankle fusion. However, alignment and balance are still mandatory for implant survival. Trajkovski and colleagues' prospective study demonstrated that satisfactory results can be achieved in patients with preoperative coronal plane varus deformity of more than 10° if alignment and balance were obtained.[1] In its surgical technique's article base on this original study, T. Daniels outlined the goals of TAR[2]:

- Achieve a balanced, stable, congruent ankle joint with plantigrade alignment of the hindfoot and forefoot.
- Place all components perpendicular to the plumb line of the body, so that all components are parallel to the floor when the patient is standing.
- Restore ankle range of motion.

[a] Centre Cheville & Pied, Clinique St Léonard, 18 rue de Béllinière, Trélazé 49800, France; [b] Pole de santé Léonard de Vinci - 1 avenue du professeur Alexandre Minkowski - 37170 Chambray les Tours, France; [c] Département de Chirurgie Osseuse, CHU-Angers, 4, rue Larrey, 49933 Angers cedex 9, France
* Corresponding author.
E-mail address: professeurjeanbrilhault@gmail.com

Foot Ankle Clin N Am 28 (2023) 833–842
https://doi.org/10.1016/j.fcl.2023.05.011
1083-7515/23/© 2023 Elsevier Inc. All rights reserved.

Although T. Daniels stated that if these goals could not be accomplished, a fusion should be considered, he mentioned that a staged procedure involving deformity correction and secondary TAR was possible and outlined the principals of this concept. More recently, Steginsky and Haddad detailed their approaches of this 2-stage procedure concept.[3] We have been successful following their recommendations.[4] We illustrate here our current approach to TAR in cavovarus deformity.

The general principle is to correct the cavovarus and ankle deformity first, then proceed with the ankle joint replacement, the lateral ligament stabilization, and the forefoot balance (adaptive cavovarus due to tibia varus deformity will not be addressed here). Ancillary procedures include plantar fascia release, release/lengthening of the posterior tibial tendon (PTT), release of the talonavicular capsule, lateral displacement calcaneal osteotomy, PTT transfer to the peroneus brevis, lateral ligament reconstruction, and dorsiflexion osteotomy of the first metatarsal bone. Occasionally hindfoot fusion or midfoot osteotomy is required. Although we favor single-stage procedures, we propose 2-stage procedures when (1) gross hindfoot deformity requires bony procedure such as double arthrodesis, triple arthrodesis, or midfoot osteotomy (**Fig. 1**); (2) gross lateral ligament instability with associated severe cavovarus deformity requires tendon transfer combined with complex lateral ligament reconstruction; (3) rigid deformity correction requires combined ancillary procedure jeopardize wound healing; and (4) there is questionable skin status that might contraindicate TAR.

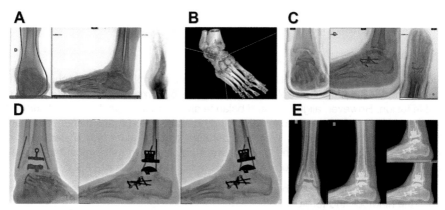

Fig. 1. Case of severe cavovarus deformity of the right foot associated with fixed varus osteoarthritis (OA) of the ankle due to postpolio syndrome (*A*). The patient underwent hindfoot fusion during childhood. Complete L5 deficiency induced a remaining drop foot. Remaining muscles were triceps 4/5, FDL 4/5, and FHL 4/5. Malunion of the Chopart joint fusion was appreciated on the computed tomography (CT) 3-dimensional (3D) reconstruction (*B*). The patient was proposed a 2-stage surgery based on the bony deformity of the foot and the muscle deficiency that both needed to be addressed before TAR surgery. After releasing the ankle joint, a dome-shaped osteotomy was performed at the Chopart joint fusion. Once realigned, a lateral ligament Evans reconstruction was performed. An FDL transfer was performed to address the drop foot and spare the FHL in order to maintain push-off. The gutter debridement and the lateral ligament reconstruction maintained the talus in a proper position, enabling to avoid cement filling of the medial gutter (*C*). TAR was performed 3 months later with prophylactic malleolar screws. One-year follow-up ankle radiographs demonstrated deformities correction as well as good range of motion (*D*). Clinical and radiological results are maintained at 4 years follow-up (*E*).

CORRECTION OF THE FOOT DEFORMITY
Cavus Deformity

If there is a substantial cavus deformity with a tight plantar fascia, a Steindler release is performed.[5] Incision is performed obliquely on the medial aspect of the heel. Fatty tissues are bluntly reflected in order to avoid injury to the medial calcaneal nerve until the medial superficial fascia is visualized. The fascia is cut in order to mobilize the abductor muscle belly dorsally and to access its deep fascia. The deep fascia is cut respecting the underlying fatty tissue in which runs the fifth toe abductor nerve. Moving plantar, fasciotomy is completed and plantar fascia is identified. Room is made around the plantar fascia to be safely sectioned with scissors from medial to lateral as far as required to correct the cavus deformity. Occasionally short muscles must be stripped from the plantar aspect of the calcaneus using a broad periosteal elevator in order to complete the deformity correction. Completion of the plantar release can be checked manually.

Correction of the forefoot remaining deformity due to a plantarflexed first metatarsal is performed after rearfoot and ankle realignment. It usually requires a dorsiflexion osteotomy of the first metatarsal bone but cuneometatarsal joint arthrodesis might be performed as well.

Adductus Deformity

If the foot can be everted to a neutral position, release of the PTT and the talonavicular capsule is usually performed through the anterior approach. If the foot cannot be everted past neutral, the PTT usually needs to be transferred to the peroneus brevis tendon (**Fig. 2**). The release is then realized through a medial incision. The PTT sheath is open, and the PTT is released from the talonavicular capsule. The talonavicular capsule is transected vertically, and a complete release of the talonavicular joint is performed including the spring ligament. Completion of the release is achieved with a blunt Cobb elevator in order to dig the talus head out of the coxa pedis complex. At the end of the procedure a passive eversion of the midfoot should be possible. If eversion of the foot cannot be achieved, fusion should be performed. If eversion is prevented by the PTT, it is released from the navicular bone and prepared for transfer.

If the foot self-aligns, no need to fix the talonavicular joint, and if not, we recommend stabilization with a K-wire or a 3.5 mm screw until soft tissues are healed (**Fig. 3**).

If a PTT transfer to the peroneus brevis is to be performed, proximal release to the PTT sheath is performed to facilitate delivery of the PTT proximally. A posteromedial incision is performed in the supramalleolar area to expose the proximal aspect of the PTT. The PTT is identified and will secondarily be pulled out from the wound for transfer.

In case of malunion of the hindfoot we perform a cylindrical osteotomy through a double anteromedial and lateral approach using a 3 mm Shannon burr. Once the osteotomy is performed, the midfoot can be everted into proper position and forefoot pronosupination balanced. Fixation is performed with lag screws and 2 locking plates, one on each foot column.

Varus Deformity

Varus deformity correction should be addressed once the ankle joint part of the varus deformity has been dealt with and if a varus heel remains.

In case of malunion of a triple hindfoot arthrodesis correction of the adductus deformity is performed first. If subtalar malunion into varus requires alignment after correction of the varus deformity at ankle level, it is obtained with a percutaneous calcaneus osteotomy, leaving the fused subtalar joint untouched.[6]

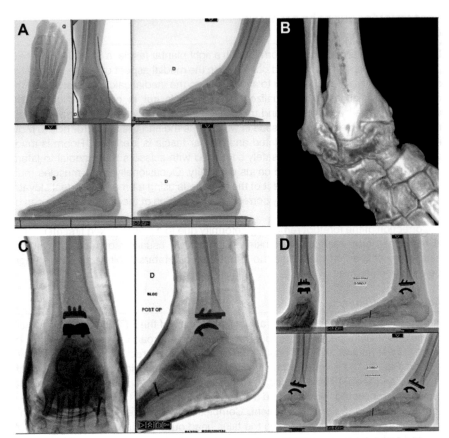

Fig. 2. Case of a right ankle OA from chronic lateral instability on congenital bilateral cavovarus feet. Preoperative imaging demonstrated a mild incongruent varus ankle deformity (*A*) with osteophyte formation on the lateral malleolus (*B*). Active eversion was limited due to peroneus brevis tendon chronic rupture. In this case we performed lateral gutter debridement with trimming of both fibula and talus; release of the talonavicular joint through a medial approach because we planned to transfer the posterior tibial tendon; and release of the medial gutter with malleolar peel of the deltoid ligament with ligament release from sustentaculum tali in order to realign the heel. A TAR was implanted with reference to the lateral tibio-fibula-talus intersection at Shenton line level. Protruding medial malleolus was trimmed to prevent impingement with the soft tissues. Lateral reconstruction was performed with a Brostrom procedure. Posterior tibial tendon transfer to the peroneus brevis distal stump was performed. Persistent forefoot pronation required a dorsiflexion oblique osteotomy of the first metatarsal bone (*C*). One year follow-up radiographs document the hypercorrection of the cavus with a slight dorsiflexed first ray at 1-year follow-up (*D*).

CORRECTION OF THE ANKLE DEFORMITY
Lateral Debridement

More often than not, osteophytes are present on the lateral aspect of the ankle, blocking the talus into varus and adduction (**Fig. 4**).[7] We therefore start laterally.

Peroneus tendon sheath is cut open anterior to the tip of the fibula. Tendons are inspected for tendinopathy, tear, or rupture.

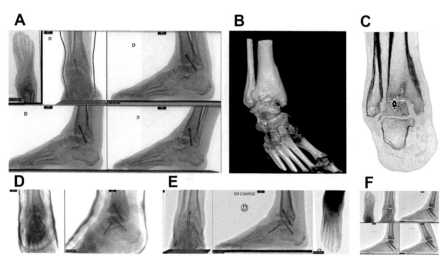

Fig. 3. Case of a bilateral arthroscopic ankle nonunion on paralytic rigid cavovarus feet due to Charcot-Marie-Tooth disease. Cavovarus foot was rigid. Tibialis posterior 4+/5 and triceps 4/5 muscle remained. Preoperative imaging demonstrated a mobile ankle nonunion and foot deformity (*A, B*). Preoperative CT documents satisfactory bone stock (*C*). The patient was proposed a 2-stage surgery based on the bony deformity of the foot and the muscle deficiency that both needed to be addressed before TAR surgery. Release of the talonavicular joint was performed through a medial approach because of the planned posterior tibial tendon transfer. Hindfoot release could not achieve limited eversion, and stabilization required arthroereisis with two 3.5 mm screw. A lateral ligament Evans type reconstruction was performed with the paralytic peroneus brevis tendon. Posterior tibial tendon was then transferred to the dorsal aspect of the foot through the interosseous membrane and split longitudinally into 2 separate arms (medial arm transferred to the anterior tibial tendon, lateral arm to the lateral cuneiform) (*D*). Second stage was at 3 months once scars were bleached and patient returned to full weight-bearing (*E*). A Salto Talaris XT TAR was implanted in order to obtain solid bone fixation through keeled implants after subtalar fusion. One-year follow-up weight-bearing ankle radiographs demonstrate a stable ankle prosthesis with complete correction of the ankle and foot deformities as well as good range of motion (*F*). A similar 2-stage procedure was performed on the left ankle the year after.

Extensor retinaculum and both anterior talofibular and calcaneofibular ligament are carefully identified and stripped off the fibula. These structures are evaluated to check whether or not a Brostrom-Gould procedure can be performed.

Debridement of the osteophytes is performed at the fibula, the body, and the lateral tubercle of the talus to clear the ankle mortise aiming for reduction of the talus on the fibula. Lateral debridement of the anterolateral plafond will be completed through the anterior approach.

Anteromedial Debridement

Anteromedial debridement is performed through a standard anterior approach. Osteophytes are resected from the tibia plafond, the medial malleolus, and the talus.

Debridement of the medial gutter is performed by removing the deep deltoid ligament debris down to the PTT sheath that is open longitudinally from the posteromedial corner of the ankle to the navicular bone.

A baby lamina spreader is positioned in the medial corner of the ankle in order to correct the intraarticular deformity and rotate the talus backward and externally to

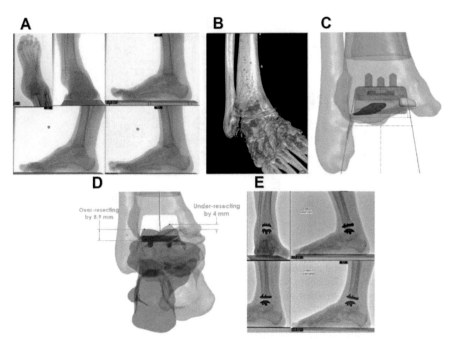

Fig. 4. Case of a bilateral ankle OA with severe incongruent varus tibiotalar deformity (*A*). Osteophyte formation in the lateral joint space was visualized on CT (*B*). Eversion was limited but possible due to peroneus brevis tear tendinopathy. A Prophecy planning was performed in this case bringing to light the dysplastic medial malleolus (*C*). Impingement between the talus and the fibula once deformity reduced is illustrated by the overlap of the talus on the fibula on the Prophecy plan (*D*). In this case we performed lateral gutter debridement with trimming of both fibula and talus; release of the talonavicular joint with release of the posterior tibial tendon through the anterior approach, and release of the medial gutter with malleolar peel of the deltoid ligament without requiring ligament release from sustentaculum tali. A hybrid TAR (Infinity tibia, InBone Talus due to the flat top talus) was implanted. Protruding anteromedial malleolus was trimmed to prevent impingement with the soft tissues. Lateral reconstruction was performed with a Brostrom procedure augmented with one-third of the peroneus brevis tendon from the tendinopathy tear debridement. Peroneus longus to brevis transfer was performed. Distal resection of the peroneus longus tendon induced a release of the forefoot pronation that reprieve the planned dorsiflexion osteotomy of the first metatarsal bone. Alignment was documented at 1-year follow-up (*E*).

achieve reduction of the talofibular joint line. If correction of the deformity cannot be achieved, subperiosteal stripping of the medial ligament is performed from the medial malleolus.[8] This technique is preferred to the medial malleolus osteotomy we performed before because we move on to fixed-bearing TAR that do not require mediolateral stabilization of the mobile insert.

Once properly positioned, the talus is fixed with 2 K-wires from the medial malleolus to evaluate repercussions on the hindfoot joints.

1. If correction of the varus deformity at the ankle induces a varus deformity of the calcaneus, the deltoid ligament is stripped from the sustentaculum tali using a curved osteotome along the medial gutter until heel realignment is obtained.
2. If not, a lateral displacement calcaneus osteotomy is performed percutaneously.[8]

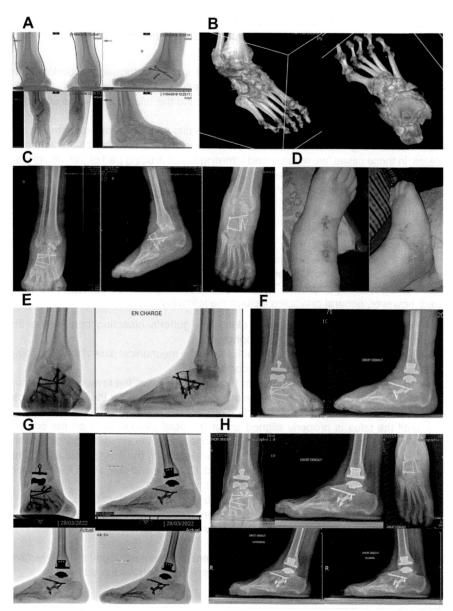

Fig. 5. Case of a severe cavovarus deformity of the right foot associated with fixed varus OA of the ankle secondary to postpolio syndrome (*A*). The patient underwent hindfoot fusion with posterior tibial tendon transfer at 30 years of age. Malunion of the Chopart joint fusion was appreciated with CT 3D reconstruction (*B*). The patient was proposed a 2-stage surgery based on the bony deformity, the lateral ligament, and wound healing issues that prevented single-stage surgery. Extensile release of the deltoid ligament was performed all the way to the calcaneus to achieve alignment of both ankle and heel. The medial ankle gap was filled with cement. Existing hardware was removed in order to perform a dome-shaped osteotomy at the level of the existing Chopart arthrodesis. Lateral ligament reconstruction was performed with an Evans type procedure using the paralyzed peroneus brevis tendon with a peroneus

3. If correction of the varus deformity at the ankle joint induces adduction, PTT is stripped from the navicular bone along with complete transection of the talonavicular capsule including the spring ligament.

If a midfoot osteotomy or fusion of the hindfoot is to be performed, it is performed at that stage of the procedure. If a 2-stage procedure is to be performed, antibiotic cement is inserted in the gap between the tibia and the talus (**Fig. 5**). The cement is allowed to cure before removing the K-wires.

Care must be taken not to let a protruding medial malleolus impinge with the soft tissues after realignment of the ankle; this is frequently the case in Takakura stage 4 ankles. In these cases, we recommend trimming the protruding part of the medial malleolus to prevent from the trestle effect on the soft tissues. The soft tissues are then closed in a standard layered fashion.

ANKLE REPLACEMENT

Fixed-bearing TAR is favored in these cases because of the intrinsic stability it provides. If a 2-stage procedure is performed, we wait until the wound scars to be bleached before doing so. Cement is usually removed without difficulty, and the ankle replacement is then performed. The TAR procedure depends on the type of implant used; however, general principles include the following:

- Rotational alignment is usually along the gutter's bisection considering the medial wear and the lateral osteophytes.
- The tibial cut is performed perpendicular to the mechanical axis of the tibia going up to any defect in the medial plafond.
- Talus is properly positioned within the ankle mortise at the level of the Shenton line, making sure there is no lateral impingement between the lateral tubercle and the fibula. If so, limited resection of the talus and/or the fibula is performed until the talus is properly aligned under the tibial plafond both on the coronal plane and the sagittal plane. Care is taken to check the sagittal alignment under fluoroscopy, making sure the sinus tarsi aligned with the mechanical axis of the tibia. Once the talus is properly positioned, it is fixed into place with K-wires, and the proximal cut of the talus dome is performed.
- The remaining procedure depends on the type of the implant used.
- Trial polyethylene thickness is chosen in order to position the talus at the Shenton line level and restore physiologic congruency of the talofibular joint line restoring the dime sign.[9]
- Ankle stability and clearance of both gutters are checked. If gutter impingement is observed, it is cleared using a 3-mm thick Shannon wedge burr.

---

longus to brevis transfer distally (C). Delayed wound healing required prolonged wound care until 6 weeks (D). Second stage was performed at 3 months postop once the scars bleached and weight-bearing resumed (E). Bone quality was good enough to avoid prophylactic malleolar screws. A Talaris TAR was implanted. Rotational alignment of the ankle and the heel was privileged over the forefoot that left 15° of adduction. Postoperative wound healing was uneventful and patient returned to full weight-bearing in a walking boot at 3 weeks (F). One-year follow-up weight-bearing ankle radiographs demonstrate a stable ankle prosthesis with complete correction of the ankle and foot deformities as well as good range of motion (G). Clinical and radiological results were maintained at 2-year follow-up (H).

LATERAL STABILIZATION

If the lateral ligaments are of good quality, a Brostrom-Gould procedure is performed. More often than not, the peroneal tendons are diseased or ruptured in these cases.

- If the peroneus brevis is ruptured, the peroneus longus is transferred to the peroneus brevis using a Pulvertaft weave technique.
- If both fibular tendons are diseased, we recommend transferring the PTT to the peroneus brevis using the same technique.

In both cases peroneus remaining stump can be used to perform a nonanatomic ligamentoplasty or to augment a Brostrom technique. If there is no lateral laxity (calcaneofibular ligament) but an anterolateral laxity involving both the ankle (anterior talofibular ligament) and the subtalar joint, we favor a Hemi-Castaing/Evans technique locking the half peroneus brevis stump in the lateral malleolus at the ligament common footprint with an interference screw. If a lateral laxity is present, we recommend a modified Chrisman-Snook technique with a subcutaneous return of the tendon graft lateral to the peroneus longus tendon to a drill hole at the origin of the calcaneofibular ligament on the calcaneus fixed with a second interference screw.[10]

FOREFOOT PRONATION

The last step of the cavovarus reconstruction requires addressing the pronation of the first metatarsal bone. The need for this procedure is detected clinically once the alignment of the ankle and rearfoot has been obtained. In case of a 2-stage procedure this last step is performed in the second stage in order to fine-tune the forefoot balance to the ankle alignment. More often than not it is addressed with a closing wedge osteotomy performed at the base of the first metatarsal. We currently perform this osteotomy percutaneously with a 2-mm Shannon burr and oblique dorsoplantar screw fixation. Less frequently the apex of the cavus deformity is at the medial cuneometatarsal joint. If so, a closing wedge arthrodesis of the medial cuneometatarsal joint is performed through an open approach. Fixation is performed with both a compression screw and a dorsomedial locking plate in order to access early weight-bearing.

All wounds are closed in layers with interrupted resorbable sutures. Suction drain is usually not used. The leg is placed into a well-padded splint. Patient is kept non–weight-bearing for 2 to 3 weeks to allow for soft tissue healing. Progressive weight-bearing with a walking boot and 2 crutches starts at 3 weeks. Full weight-bearing if pain free is authorized at 6 weeks. A walking boot is maintained until 9 weeks if TAR is performed, until second stage if a 2-stage procedure is planned. Second stage is performed once bony procedures are healed and wound scares are bleached, which usually occurs at 12 weeks postoperatively.

CLINICS CARE POINTS

- Prognostic is more about alignment and balance obtained at the end of surgery than about preoperative deformity.
- If alignment and balance cannot be obtained consider staging or fusing.
- Lateral debridement should be performed first in order to make place for talus relocation in the ankle and to prevent over-releasing the medial ligament complex.
- Medial release involves both malleolar peel and deltoid release for the sustentaculum tali in order to prevent the calcaneus to shift medially.

- Posterior tibial muscle is the deforming force here. Consider releasing the tendon from the navicular bone and transfer to the peroneus brevis tendon it is as efficient as any lateral ligament reconstruction to prevent varus instability.
- Keep in mind the Tanaka medial malleolus ware when aligning the TAR in rotation.
- Shenton line is the beacon of joint line level.
- Don't forget to address forefoot pronation with a dorsiflexion first column procedure before calling it over.

DISCLOSURE

J.M. Brilhault: Royalty Bearing Surgeon, Newclip Technics, Inc.; Consultant, Newclip Technics, Inc. and Stryker Inc. G. Auboyneau: nothing to disclose. L. Ronny: Consultant, Johnson & Johnson, Inc. and Newclip Technics, Inc.

REFERENCES

1. Trajkovski T, Pinsker E, Cadden A, et al. Outcomes of ankle arthroplasty with preoperative coronal-plane varus deformity of 10° or greater. J Bone Joint Surg Am 2013;95(15):1382–8.
2. Daniels TR. Surgical Technique for Total Ankle Arthroplasty in Ankles with Preoperative Coronal Plane Varus Deformity of 10° or Greater. JBJS Essent Surg Tech 2014;3(4):e22.
3. Steginsky B, Haddad SL. Two-Stage Varus Correction. Foot Ankle Clin 2019; 24(2):281–304.
4. Boble M, Le Nail LR, Brilhault J. Impact of preoperative varus on ankle replacement survival. Orthop Traumatol Surg Res 2022;108(7):103390.
5. Steindler A. The treatment of pes cavus (hollow claw foot). Arch Surg 1921;2(2): 325–37.
6. Brilhault J. Calcaneal osteotomy for hindfoot deformity. Orthop Traumatol Surg Res 2022;108(1s):103121.
7. Seki H, Ogihara N, Kokubo T, et al. Visualization and quantification of the degenerative pattern of the distal tibia and fibula in unilateral varus ankle osteoarthritis. Sci Rep 2021;11(1):21628.
8. Bonnin M, Judet T, Colombier JA, et al. Midterm results of the Salto Total Ankle Prosthesis. Clin Orthop Relat Res 2004;424:6–18.
9. Harper MC, Keller TS. A radiographic evaluation of the tibiofibular syndesmosis. Foot Ankle Int 1989;10(3):156–60.
10. Acevedo JI, Myerson MS. Modification of the Chrisman-Snook technique. Foot Ankle Int 2000;21(2):154–5.

Supramalleolar Osteotomies in Cavovarus Foot Deformity
Why Patient-Specific Instruments Make a Difference

Arne Burssens, MD, PhD[a],*, Bernhard Devos Bevernage, MD[a,b],
Kristian Buedts, MD[c]

KEYWORDS

- Supramalleolar osteotomy • Cavovarus deformity • Hindfoot alignment
- Weight-bearing CT • Patient-specific instrumentation

KEY POINTS

- Supramalleolar osteotomy enables deformity correction of the ankle joint in cavovarous foot deformity.
- Most supramalleolar osteotomies are currently planned preoperatively on 2-dimensional weight-bearing radiographs and executed peroperatively using free-hand techniques.
- This article encompasses 3-dimensional (3D) planning and printing techniques based on weight-bearing computed tomography images and patient-specific instruments (PSIs) to correct ankle varus deformities.
- An overview of 3D planning software and PSI design for both a closing wedge and dome-shaped supramalleolar osteotomy will be presented.
- These techniques have the potential to overcome the shortcomings of plain weight-bearing radiographs and mitigate the technical drawbacks of free-hand supramalleolar osteotomies.

INTRODUCTION

Supramalleolar osteotomy (SMOT) enables deformity correction of the ankle joint and is associated with improvement of pain and function in the short term and long term.[1-10] Despite these beneficial results, the amount of surgical correction is challenging to titrate and the procedure remains technically demanding.[11,12] At present, the amount of deformity correction is determined on plain radiographs (RX) using

[a] Department of Orthopaedics, Ghent University Hospital, Corneel Heymanslaan 10, Ghent 9000, Belgium; [b] Department of Orthopaedics, Foot and Ankle Institute, Avenue Ariane 5, Brussels 1000, Belgium; [c] Department of Orthopaedics, ZNA Middelheim, Lindendreef 1, Antwerp 2020, Belgium
* Corresponding author.
E-mail address: arne.burssens@ugent.be

Foot Ankle Clin N Am 28 (2023) 843–856
https://doi.org/10.1016/j.fcl.2023.06.002
1083-7515/23/© 2023 Elsevier Inc. All rights reserved.

mathematical calculations.[10,13] However, this medical imaging modality is subjected to measurement errors of the ankle joint alignment caused by variance in patient positioning (**Fig. 1A, B**).[14] Moreover, it has also been demonstrated that the measurement of ankle joint alignment depends on using short or long radiographic images of the tibia.[15] Another limitation of plain radiographs is the 2-dimensional (2D) projection of ankle joint deformity, which is often 3-dimensional (3D) in nature.[16–18]

The recent advent of weight-bearing conebeam CT (WBCT) imaging overcomes the aforementioned shortcomings by correcting rotational errors based on postimaging reconstructions, avoiding superposition due to circumferential imaging of the osseous structures and generating 3D models of ankle deformity during physiologic stance.[17,19–27] Recent technical advancements in patient-specific guides in the lower limb based on 3D printing[28] have also mitigated some of the shortcoming related to the free-hand osteotomies (eg, unequal wedge size; see **Fig. 1A, B**). However, most of these studies combined alignment calculations on weight-bearing radiographs and generated the patient-specific guides non–weight-bearing CT. Hereby, the limitations of plain radiographs in deformity planning remain present and the full potential of 3D imaging does not get unlocked.

Only a paucity of literature is available that used 3D WBCT imaging to perform both the deformity planning and design of patient-specific guides.[29,30]

For this reason, the goal of this article is to go deeper in this technique and provide a stepwise approach in performing a 3D preoperative planning and design of a patient-specific guide for patients with ankle varus deformity.

PREOPERATIVE PLANNING

At our department, 2 types of supramalleolar osteotomies are preferred for ankle varus deformity: a lateral distal tibia closing wedge SMOT and a dome-shaped SMOT.

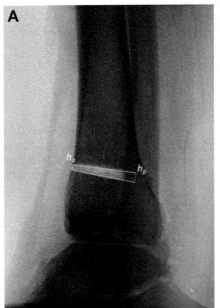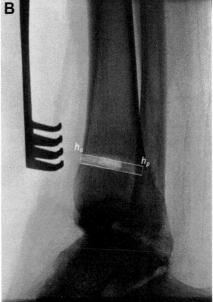

Fig. 1. Example of an unequal wedge size noted during a free-hand lateral distal tibia closing wedge osteotomy (*A*) Before correction: $h_a < h_p$ (*B*) After correction: $h_a = h_p$.

Although we acknowledge all benefits from a medial distal tibia opening wedge SMOT, we wanted to elude potential downsides from this type of SMOT such as stretch on the medial soft tissues (including the posterior tibial tendon) and the need for an additional bone graft.[31]

In case of congruent ankle varus deformity, we will opt for a lateral distal tibia-closing wedge SMOT if the wedge size calculation is ≤ 8 *mm* and dome-shaped SMOT if the wedge size calculation is >8 *mm*. In case of a dyscongruent ankle varus deformity, we will opt for a lateral distal tibia-closing wedge SMOT combined with inframalleolar procedures.

Lateral Distal Tibia-Closing Wedge SMOT

a. Two-dimensional weight-bearing RX planning

Preoperative planning of ankle varus deformity correction has classically been performed at our department on weight-bearing anterioposterior (AP) radiographs obtained with a Meary incidence (**Fig. 2**).[32,33] This radiographic imaging method requires the feet positioned "parallel" to the axis of the second metatarsal. The outline of the hindfoot is marked with radiopaque metal reference points, at the height of both malleoli. The radiographic beam is positioned horizontally and focused on the center of the ankle. The tibial anterior surface (TAS) angle and tibio talar surface (TTS) angle (see **Fig. 2**A) were respectively defined by intersecting the best-fitted longitudinal tibial shaft axis with the axis of the tibial plafond and talar dome in the coronal plane (TAS/TTS; normal range, 93.3 ± 3.2/91.5 ± 1.2° of valgus).[15,34] The talar tilt (TT) angle can be determined by the difference between the TAS and TTS angle (TT; normal range, 0°–4° of varus).[35] The hindfoot angle (HA) was determined according to the method of Méary by intersecting the best-fitted longitudinal tibial shaft axis with the axis of the hindfoot at the superior surface of the talus and center between both metal reference points (HA: 3°–6° of valgus).[33,36,37]

After determining these angles, we translate the distal tibial surface axis, approximately 2.5 cm proximal (see **Fig. 2**B, TAS'). This simulates our first osteotomy cut, which is preferably just above the ankle syndesmosis to avoid ligamentous injuries.[38] Next, we determine our TAS" that we want to achieve postoperatively in the normal range of 93.3 ± 3.2° of valgus (see **Fig. 2**C). The distance *h*, measured on the lateral contour of the distal tibia between the original (TAS') and projected position (TAS"), will constitute the seize of our wedge. The angle *α* of this wedge will inform us on the magnitude of deformity correction relative to the tibial axis that can be expected after SMOT (see **Fig. 2**D). If *α* exceeds the varus HA by ≥ 3°, then the HA will be brought back to its normal range and an additional calcaneal osteotomy will most likely not be required.

b. Three-dimensional weight-bearing CT planning

At our department, we prefer to obtain a weight-bearing conebeam CT to generate our 3D model of the cavovarus deformity (**Fig. 3**A, B). Many software modules are available to create from 2D CT slices a 3D structure. An important part of this process is the segmentation tools that allow to designate each osseous component (tibia, fibula, and talus) in the 3D model. As an example, we present 2 types of software modules that can be used: **Fig. 4**A demonstrating Disior Bonelogic (Paragon28, Denver, US) and **Fig. 4**B depicting Mimics combined with 3-matic (Mataralise, Leuven, BE).

We often start our 3D segmentation process in Disior Bonelogic, which has the advantage to offer semiautomated segmentation and measurement tools. This 3D model is exported as a stereolithography file an import in Mimics to analyze it against

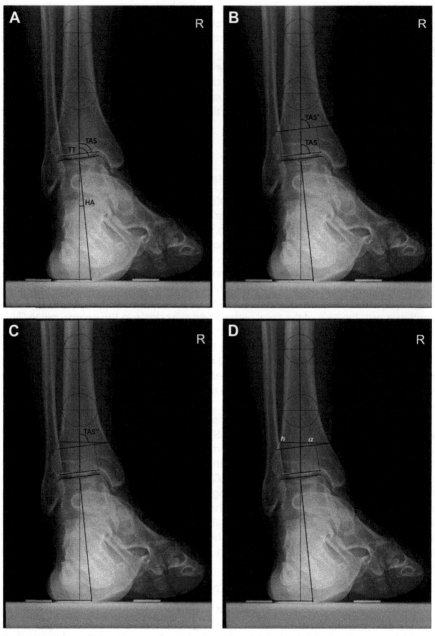

Fig. 2. Overview of the 2D preoperative planning of lateral distal tibia closing wedge osteotomy (A) Measurement of the coronal ankle and hindfoot alignment (B) Translation of the TAS angle 2.5 cm above the ankle joint line (TAS') (C) The desired TAS" is determined (D) The wedge size (h) to obtain TAS" is calculated.

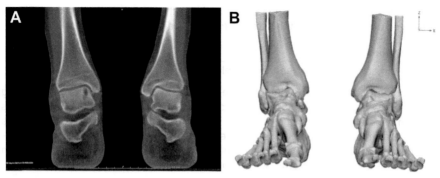

Fig. 3. Weight-bearing CT scan of a patient with ankle varus deformity and a medial talar cyst (*A*) 2D CT slices (*B*) 3D CT reconstruction.

the single CT slices. After this step, the model is export in 3-matic to perform the design of the patient-specific instrumentation. When this process would be too time-consuming or complex, it is also possible to use platforms provided by the industry to upload the Digital Imaging and Communications in Medicine (DICOM) images of the weight-bearing CT scan, which will be used to design patient-specific instrumentation in conjunction with the hardware. In this light, we recently started to work with the Orthopedics Newgen Excellence (ONE) platform provided by Newclip (Nantes, FR). On the platform, the surgeon can upload the DICOM images of the weight-bearing RX and CT scan and select the desired amount of deformity correction as

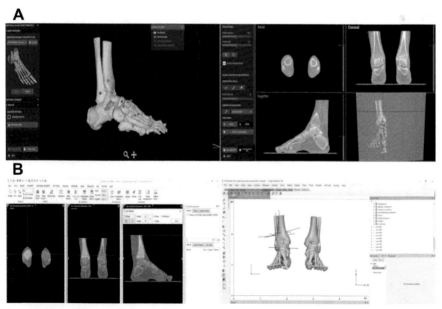

Fig. 4. Overview of 3D software modules (*A*) Disior Bonelogic (Paragon28, Denver, US) software allows semiautomated segmentation and measurements after selecting the correct osseous structures (*B*) Mimics combined with 3-matic (Matarialise, Leuven, BE) software allows manual segmentation and uses computer-aided design operations to calculate axes and angles.

well as the osteotomy type. A preoperative plan with patient-specific guide design is generated and proposed to the surgeon for approval (**Fig. 5A**).

Dome-Shaped SMOT

a. Two-dimensional weight-bearing RX planning

In correspondence to the preoperative planning of the lateral distal tibia-closing wedge SMOT, an AP weight-bearing radiograph of the ankle with Méary view is used. In general, the TAS of the deformity is measured and the desired postoperative TAS is determined. The difference between both is the angular amount of the deformity correction (α). As a general rule of thumb, we calculate that 1 mm of translation in the dome-shaped osteotomy, which corresponds to 1° of angular correction.[12]

a. Three-dimensional weight-bearing CT planning

Similar to the preoperative planning of a lateral distal tibia-closing wedge SMOT, a weight-bearing conebeam CT is obtained to generate a 3D model of the cavovarus deformity. The 3D model is imported in 3-matic (Materialise), and computer-aided design (CAD) operations are used to compose a circle with a radius (r) of 3 to 4 cm, the center of the ankle joint is set as the center of the circle. Next, a guide is fitted on the surface and contours of the distal tibia. The drill holes are positioned parallel with the outer edge of the circle. Using a software function called "cut plane," the distal fragment of dome-shaped osteotomy can be rotated until the desired amount of correction is achieved. Next, a second guide is generated that matches with the position of the correct distal tibia. This holds both fragments proximal and distal from the osteotomy in place, so that a plate fixation can be easily applied, without loosening

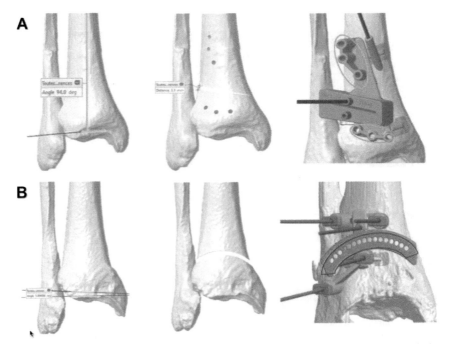

Fig. 5. Overview of a preoperative planning and patient-specific guide design provided on the ONE platform of Newclip Technics (Nantes, FR) (A) Closing wedge SMOT (B) Dome-shaped SMOT.

the reduction.[30] Similar to the guide design of closing wedge SMOT, we started to use the online platform provide by Newclip (Nantes, FR) to generate the preoperative planning and patient-specific instrument (PSI; see **Fig. 5B**).

SURGICAL TECHNIQUE

Surgery was performed under combined anesthesia containing a popliteal nerve block and subsequent general anesthesia. The patient was positioned supine and sandbag was placed underneath thigh to obtain a straight position of the foot. A pillow was positioned underneath the lower leg to allow fluoroscopic images in the lateral view. Disinfectant draping procedures are used, and a high thigh tourniquet is inflated at 270 mm Hg. A direct anterior approach is performed to expose the tibia for both the closing wedge and dome-shaped osteotomies.

Lateral Distal Tibia-Closing Wedge SMOT

Free-hand procedure

A 2.00 mm k-wire is drilled from the medial flange of the distal tibia as entry point to the exit point, just above the ankle syndesmosis (**Fig. 6**A–F). The osteotomy is initiated using a TPX motor (Strycker, MI, US) and performed colinear with the k-wire. Once this cut has been been executed, the distance *h* from the reoperative planning is marked on the bone. A second osteotomy cut is performed from this point toward the medial hinge. Once the wedge is completed, it is left in situ to leave some stability before performing the fibula osteotomy. A lateral fibula approach is preferred, and a lateral

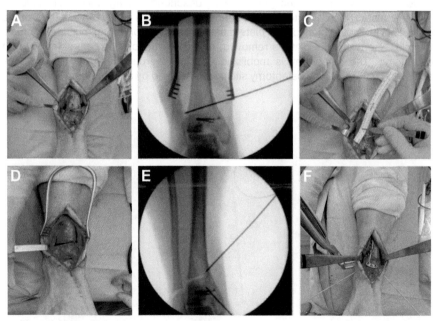

Fig. 6. Sequential approach of a free-hand closing wegde SMOT by surgeon (AB) in a patient with ankle varus deformity. (*A*) Placement of a 2 mm k-wire. (*B*) Image intensifier verifies that the k-wire starts perpendicular on the medial flenge of the distal tibia and enters suprasyndesmotic on the lateral side. (*C*) Measurement of wedge size. (*D*) Removal of the calculated bone wedge. (*E*) Verification on image intensifier. (*F*) Closing of the osteotomy by use of Hintermann compressor and plate fixation.

closing wedge is performed at the height of the distal tibia osteotomy. After the fibula osteotomy, the wedge at the distal tibia osteotomy is removed and 2 × 2.00mm crossed k-wires are being positioned in place before the closing of the osteotomy. This step is performed manually by applying a lateral force of the heel; gentleness is key, otherwise the medial bone hinge has the risk to break. When the osteotomy has difficulties to close, the author prefers to use the Hintermann compressor (Integra LifeSciences, Plainsboro, NJ, US). This elegant device allows a gradual compression/closing of the osteotomy and even in case of breakage at the level of the hinge, the proximal and distal tibia fragments are kept in place. After closing of the osteotomy, the 2 k-wires are drilled through the lateral cortex to preliminary fixate the osteotomy. Afterward, a definite fixation is performed using an anterolateral Activmotion S Distal Tibia Osteotomy plate (Newclip).

- PSI procedure

After exposing the distal tibia, the patient-specific guide can only be positioned in the correct place based on the osseous contours. This corresponds to a firm and stable attachment on the distal tibia. K-wires of 2 mm were applied in dedicated sleeves of the guide to maintain a correct position on the distal tibia (**Fig. 7**A). The cutting length on the saw can be marked by steristrip (**Fig. 7**B).

Dome-Shaped SMOT

Free-hand procedure
Following exposition of the distal tibia, a dome-shaped supramalleolar osteotomy was performed based on the technique previously described by Wagner and colleagues.[12] A 4-hole plate (Tibiaxys, Integra LifeSciences) is fixed by a screw at the center of the distal tibia but not tightened. The plate is used as a guide for drilling multiple bicortical tunnels. Afterward, the plate is removed, and the osteotomy is completed with an osteotome. The osteotomy is mobilized until an overcorrection of the TAS was achieved by 2° to 3°. The osteotomy site is compressed by a Hintermann compressor

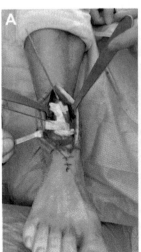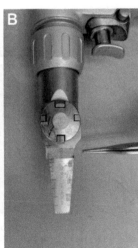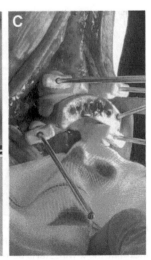

Fig. 7. Peroperative use of the patient-specific guides. (*A*) PSI in lateral closing SMOT. (*B*) Marking the saw length based on the preoperative plan using a steristrip. (*C*) PSI in dome-shaped SMOT.

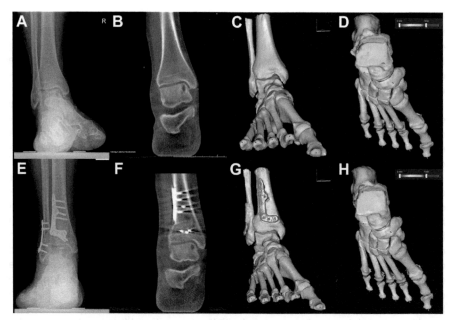

Fig. 8. Preoperative versus postoperative closing wedge SMOT correction (*A*) Preop weight-bearing 2D x-ray. (*B*) Preop weight-bearing 2D CT. (*C*) Preop weight-bearing 3D CT. (*D*) Preop distance map on weight-bearing 3D CT demonstrating lower color code on the lateral compartment of the ankle (*blue*) (*E*) Postop weight-bearing 2D x-ray. (*F*) Postop weight-bearing 2D CT. (*G*) Post weight-bearing 3D CT (*H*) Postop weight-bearing 3D CT with distance map demonstrating an equal distribution of the color code (*green*).

(Integra LifeSciences). A subsequent stabilization was performed by 2 angular stable plates (Tibiaxys, Integra LifeSciences, Princeton, NJ, USA).

Patient-specific instrument procedure
Once the distal tibia is exposed, the patient-specific guide can only be fitted in the correct position based on the osseous contours. This can be noticed by a firm and stable attachment on the distal tibia. K-wires of 2 mm were applied in dedicated sleeves of the guide to maintain the correct position on the distal tibia. Subsequently, a 2.7-mm drill guide was used to drill the holes in the remaining sleeves to obtain the dome-shaped pattern of the osteotomy. After removal of the guide, the remaining bone attachments are then manually removed with a small chisel and smoothened with a small saw blade. Afterward, the reduction guide is applied and fixed with K-wires in the correct position. Subsequently, the obtained osteotomy is stabilized by an anterior Activmotion S Distal Tibia Osteotomy plate (Newclip) and confirmed on AP and lateral fluoroscopic control. The final step involves fixing the fibula at its correct length. Either cortical screws or plate and screws were used to perform the fixation, depending on the achieved stability. Postoperatively, all patients were immobilized in a non–weight-bearing cast for 6 weeks. After bone healing was seen on a standard x-ray, full weight-bearing was allowed, and physical therapy was started.

SUMMARY

Fundamental rules on the principals of deformity correction have been constituted in a previous study.[39] However, some of these corrections are based on rather complex mathematical calculations.[40] For this reason, we often simplify these mathematical formulas to make them more applicable to our clinical practice but this occurs at cost of some inaccuracy. Aside from these preoperative planning inaccuracies, we tend to perform preoperatively most of osteotomies free-hand, which also induces a certain degree of inaccuracy. These shortcomings call for improvement in our preoperative planning and peroperative execution of supramalleolar osteotomies.

Fortunately, we are at dawn of a new area, where the bond between biomechanical engineers and orthopedic surgeons has flourished to a high level of scientific exchange and excellence.[41] Aside from these continuous collaborations, 3D software modules have become more user friendly for clinical purposes and 3D print technology has gained a widespread usage.[42–50]

This article demonstrated how both 3D planning and printing can be applied for correction of ankle varus deformity (**Fig. 8A–H**). We perceive this technology to overcome the aforementioned shortcomings of plain weight-bearing radiographs and that it mitigates the technical drawbacks of free-hand osteotomies. Compared with the literature, we found only a paucity of studies using these combined technologies in correction of ankle varus deformity.[29,30,51,52] van Raaij and colleagues,[51] Faict[53] and colleagues, and Ma and colleagues[29] used a 2-step 3D-guided approach for the correction of ankle varus deformity and demonstrated only a minimal postoperative deviation from the desired correction. Wang and colleagues[52] used a similar approach but took the comparison a step further and demonstrated that the 3D-guided patient-specific approach is superior compared with the conventional free-hand technique for supramalleolar osteotomies, both regarding clinical as well as radiographical outcome. However, despite providing promising results on the short term and midterm, all these studies were devoid of long-term results. Evenmore, although superior accuracy of patient-specific guides for osteotomy over free-hand osteotomies has been demonstrated,[54] this did not result in a clear clinical benefit for knee osteotomies.[55]

Nevertheless, we should strive to continue our endeavor in this field of supramalleolar osteotomies based on the superior short-term and midterm results.[29,30,51,52] Moreover, it could also be postulated that a higher degree of accuracy in an ankle osteotomy could be more impactful then in a knee osteotomy because the ankle has a smaller surface area and still has to carry the same amount of load as the knee. Future studies should also focus on including the soft tissues during the preoperative planning and on the impact of SMOT relative the adjacent articulations of the ankle joint.[56,57]

Ultimately, this might aid in titrating the amount SMOT correction in respect to a certain degree of alignment chance in the adjacent joints, determine which postoperative position is most beneficial to optimize patient reported outcomes (PROMs) and indicate when inframalleolar procedures are required in conjunction to a supramalleolar osteotomy.[58]

CLINICS CARE POINTS

- Supramalleolar osteotomy enables correction of the ankle varus deformity and is associated with improvement of pain and function in the short term and long term.

- Most supramalleolar osteotomies are currently planned preoperatively on 2D weight-bearing radiographs and executed peroperatively using free-hand techniques.

- A potential pitfall of performing a preoperative planning on 2D weight-bearing radiographs is to underestimate the magnitude of a 3D ankle deformity.

- A potential pitfall of performing free-hand supramalleolar osteotomies is to have the osteotomy plane in a different direction, which might interfere with the wedge or dome-shaped correction.
- As a pearl 3D planning and printing techniques based on weight-bearing CT images and PSIs to correct ankle varus deformities are presented in this article.
- These techniques have the potential to overcome the shortcomings of plain weight-bearing radiographs and mitigate the technical drawbacks of free-hand supramalleolar osteotomies.

DISCLOSURE

A. Burssens performed a consultancy for Curvebeam LLC, B. Devos Bevernage performed a consultancy for Integra LifeSciences and K. Buedts performed a consultancy for Newclip Technics.

ACKNOWLEDGMENTS

The authors acknowledge the valuable help of Loïc Raes, BMSc in generating several 3D models and Mrs Thérèse Rogiers for her kind assistance during the supramalleolar osteotomy surgeries.

REFERENCES

1. Takakura Y, Tanaka Y, Kumai T, et al. Low tibial osteotomy for osteoarthritis of the ankle. Results of a new operation in 18 patients. The Journal of bone and joint surgery British 1995;77(1):50–4.
2. Hintermann B, Knupp M, Barg A. Supramalleolar osteotomies for the treatment of ankle arthritis. J Am Acad Orthop Surg 2016;24(7):424–32.
3. Knupp M, Hintermann B. Treatment of asymmetric arthritis of the ankle joint with supramalleolar osteotomies. Foot Ankle Int 2012;33(3):250–2.
4. Lee W-C, Moon J-S, Lee K, et al. Indications for supramalleolar osteotomy in patients with ankle osteoarthritis and varus deformity. JBJS 2011;93(13):1243–8.
5. Stamatis ED, Cooper PS, Myerson MS. Supramalleolar osteotomy for the treatment of distal tibial angular deformities and arthritis of the ankle joint. Foot Ankle Int 2003;24(10):754–64.
6. Hintermann B, Ruiz R, Barg A. Novel double osteotomy technique of distal tibia for correction of asymmetric varus osteoarthritic ankle. Foot Ankle Int 2017; 38(9):970–81.
7. Ahn T-K, Yi Y, Cho J-H, et al. A cohort study of patients undergoing distal tibial osteotomy without fibular osteotomy for medial ankle arthritis with mortise widening. J Bone Joint Surg Am 2015;97(5):381–8.
8. Mann HA, Filippi J, Myerson MS. Intra-articular opening medial tibial wedge osteotomy (plafond-plasty) for the treatment of intra-articular varus ankle arthritis and instability. Foot Ankle Int 2012;33(4):255–61.
9. Lim J-W, Eom J-S, Kang SJ, et al. The Effect of Supramalleolar Osteotomy without Marrow Stimulation for Medial Ankle Osteoarthritis: Second-Look Arthroscopic Evaluation of 29 Ankles. J Bone Joint Surg Am 2021;103(19):1844–51.
10. Barg A, Saltzman CL. Single-stage supramalleolar osteotomy for coronal plane deformity. Curr Rev Musculoskelet Med 2014;7(4):277–91.
11. Colin F, Gaudot F, Odri G, et al. Supramalleolar osteotomy: techniques, indications and outcomes in a series of 83 cases. J Orthop Traumatol: Surgery & Research 2014;100(4):413–8.

12. Wagner P, Colin F, Hintermann B. Distal Tibia Dome Osteotomy. Tech Foot Ankle Surg 2014;13(2):103–7.

13. Warnock KM, Johnson BD, Wright JB, et al. Calculation of the opening wedge for a low tibial osteotomy. Foot Ankle Int 2004;25(11):778–82.

14. Barg A, Amendola RL, Henninger HB, et al. Influence of ankle position and radiographic projection angle on measurement of supramalleolar alignment on the anteroposterior and hindfoot alignment views. Foot Ankle Int 2015;36(11):1352–61.

15. Stufkens SA, Barg A, Bolliger L, et al. Measurement of the medial distal tibial angle. Foot Ankle Int 2011;32(3):288–93.

16. Benthien RA, Myerson MS. Supramalleolar osteotomy for ankle deformity and arthritis. Foot Ankle Clin 2004;9(3):475–87.

17. Richter M, de Cesar Netto C, Lintz F, et al. The Assessment of Ankle Osteoarthritis with Weight-Bearing Computed Tomography. Foot Ankle Clin 2022;27(1):13–36.

18. Bernasconi A, Cooper L, Lyle S, et al. Pes cavovarus in Charcot-Marie-Tooth compared to the idiopathic cavovarus foot: a preliminary weightbearing CT analysis. Foot Ankle Surg 2021;27(2):186–95.

19. Barg A, Bailey T, Richter M, et al. Weightbearing Computed Tomography of the Foot and Ankle: Emerging Technology Topical Review. Foot Ankle Int 2018; 39(3):376–86.

20. Lintz F, de Cesar Netto C, Barg A, et al. Weight-bearing cone beam CT scans in the foot and ankle. EFORT open reviews 2018;3(5):278–86.

21. Richter M, Seidl B, Zech S, et al. PedCAT for 3D-imaging in standing position allows for more accurate bone position (angle) measurement than radiographs or CT. Foot Ankle Surg 2014;20(3):201–7.

22. Burssens A, Peeters J, Buedts K, et al. Measuring hindfoot alignment in weight bearing CT: a novel clinical relevant measurement method. Foot Ankle Surg 2016;22(4):233–8.

23. Burssens A, Van Herzele E, Leenders T, et al. Weightbearing CT in normal hindfoot alignment—presence of a constitutional valgus? Foot Ankle Surg 2018;24(3): 213–8.

24. Bernasconi A, Cooper L, Lyle S, et al. Intraobserver and interobserver reliability of cone beam weightbearing semi-automatic three-dimensional measurements in symptomatic pes cavovarus. Foot Ankle Surg 2020;26(5):564–72.

25. Lintz F, Welck M, Bernasconi A, et al. 3D biometrics for hindfoot alignment using weightbearing CT. Foot Ankle Int 2017;38(6):684–9.

26. Zhang JZ, Lintz F, Bernasconi A, et al. 3D biometrics for hindfoot alignment using weightbearing computed tomography. Foot Ankle Int 2019;40(6):720–6.

27. Burssens ABM, Buedts K, Barg A, et al. Is Lower-limb Alignment Associated with Hindfoot Deformity in the Coronal Plane? A Weightbearing CT Analysis. Clin Orthop Relat Res 2020;478(1):154–68.

28. Aman ZS, DePhillipo NN, Peebles LA, et al. Improved Accuracy of Coronal Alignment Can Be Attained Using 3D-Printed Patient-Specific Instrumentation for Knee Osteotomies: A Systematic Review of Level III and IV Studies. Arthrosc J Arthrosc Relat Surg 2022;38(9):2741–58.

29. Ma XL, Ma JX, Zhao XW, et al. Intra-articular opening wedge osteotomy for varus ankle arthritis with computer-assisted planning and patient-specific surgical guides: a retrospective case series. BMC Musculoskelet Disord 2022;23(1).

30. Faict S, Burssens A, Van Oevelen A, et al. Correction of ankle varus deformity using patient-specific dome-shaped osteotomy guides designed on weight-bearing CT: a pilot study. Arch Orthop Trauma Surg 2023;143(2):791-799.

31. Hintermann B, Ruiz R. Joint Preservation Strategies for Managing Varus Ankle Deformities. Foot Ankle Clin 2022;27(1):37-56.

32. Meary R, Filipe G, Aubriot J, et al. Functional study of a double arthrodesis of the foot. Rev Chir Orthop Reparatrice Appar Mot 1977;63(4):345–59.

33. Dagneaux L, Moroney P, Maestro M. Reliability of hindfoot alignment measurements from standard radiographs using the methods of Meary and Saltzman. Foot Ankle Surg 2019;25(2):237–41.

34. Inman VTSJ. Inman's joints of the ankle. 2nd edition. Baltimore: Wiliams and Wilkins; 1991.

35. Cox J, Hewes TF. Normal" talar tilt angle. Clin Orthop Relat Res 1979;140:37–41.

36. Neri T, Barthelemy R, Tourné Y. Radiologic analysis of hindfoot alignment: comparison of Méary, long axial, and hindfoot alignment views. J Orthop Traumatol: Surgery & Research 2017;103(8):1211–6.

37. Tourné Y, Mabit C. Lateral ligament reconstruction procedures for the ankle. J Orthop Traumatol: Surgery & Research 2017;103(1):S171–81.

38. Nha KW, Lee SH, Rhyu IJ, et al. Safe zone for medial open-wedge supramalleolar osteotomy of the ankle: a cadaveric study. Foot Ankle Int 2016;37(1):102–8.

39. Paley D, Tetsworth K. Mechanical axis deviation of the lower limbs. Preoperative planning of uniapical angular deformities of the tibia or femur. Clin Orthop Relat Res 1992;280:48–64.

40. Sangeorzan BP, Judd RP, Sangeorzan BJ. Mathematical analysis of single-cut osteotomy for complex long bone deformity. J Biomech 1989;22(11–12):1271–8.

41. de Cesar Netto C. Foreword: Translational Research in Orthopedic Foot and Ankle Surgery. Foot Ankle Clin 2023;28(1):xv–xvi.

42. Burssens A, Barg A, van Ovost E, et al. The hind- and midfoot alignment computed after a medializing calcaneal osteotomy using a 3D weightbearing CT. Int J Comput Assist Radiol Surg 2019;14(8):1439–47.

43. Burssens A, Peeters J, Peiffer M, et al. Reliability and correlation analysis of computed methods to convert conventional 2D radiological hindfoot measurements to a 3D setting using weightbearing CT. Int J Comput Assist Radiol Surg 2018;13(12):1999–2008.

44. Burssens A, Susdorf R, Krahenbuhl N, et al. Supramalleolar Osteotomy for Ankle Varus Deformity Alters Subtalar Joint Alignment. Foot Ankle Int 2022;43(9):1194–203.

45. Burssens A, Vermue H, Weinberg M, et al. Three-dimensional correction of fibular hemimelia using a computer-assisted planning : technical report and literature review. Acta Orthop Belg 2020;86(3):383–90.

46. Krahenbuhl N, Kvarda P, Susdorf R, et al. Assessment of Progressive Collapsing Foot Deformity Using Semiautomated 3D Measurements Derived From Weightbearing CT Scans. Foot Ankle Int 2022;43(3):363–70.

47. Kvarda P, Krahenbuhl N, Susdorf R, et al. High Reliability for Semiautomated 3D Measurements Based on Weightbearing CT Scans. Foot Ankle Int 2022;43(1):91–5.

48. Peiffer M, Belvedere C, Clockaerts S, et al. Three-dimensional displacement after a medializing calcaneal osteotomy in relation to the osteotomy angle and hindfoot alignment. Foot Ankle Surg 2020;26(1):78–84.

49. Peiffer M, Burssens A, Duquesne K, et al. Personalised statistical modelling of soft tissue structures in the ankle. Comput Methods Progr Biomed 2022;218:106701.

50. Peiffer M, Duquesne K, Van Oevelen A, et al. Validation of a personalized ligament-constraining discrete element framework for computing ankle joint contact mechanics. Comput Methods Progr Biomed 2023;231:107366.

51. van Raaij T, van der Wel H, Beldman M, et al. Two-Step 3D-Guided Supramalleolar Osteotomy to Treat Varus Ankle osteoarthritis. Foot Ankle Int 2022;43(7): 937–41.

52. Wang CG, Yu DJ, Xu C, et al. Simulated operation combined with patient-specific instrumentation technology is superior to conventional technology for supramalleolar osteotomy: a retrospective comparative study. Am J Tourism Res 2021; 13(6):6087–97.

53. Faict S, Burssens A, Van Oevelen A, et al. Correction of ankle varus deformity using patient-specific dome-shaped osteotomy guides designed on weight-bearing CT: a pilot study. Arch Orthop Trauma Surg 2021;1–9.

54. Sys G, Eykens H, Lenaerts G, et al. Accuracy assessment of surgical planning and three-dimensional-printed patient-specific guides for orthopaedic osteotomies. Proc Inst Mech Eng H 2017;231(6):499–508.

55. Abdelhameed MA, Yang CZ, AlMaeen BN, et al. No benefits of knee osteotomy patient's specific instrumentation in experienced surgeon hands. Knee Surg Sports Traumatol Arthrosc 2022. https://doi.org/10.1007/s00167-022-07288-6.

56. Treppo S, Koepp H, Quan EC, et al. Comparison of biomechanical and biochemical properties of cartilage from human knee and ankle pairs. J Orthop Res 2000; 18(5):739–48.

57. Dibbern KN, Li S, Vivtcharenko V, et al. Three-Dimensional Distance and Coverage Maps in the Assessment of Peritalar Subluxation in Progressive Collapsing Foot Deformity. Foot Ankle Int 2021. 1071100720983227.

58. Hung M, Baumhauer JF, Latt LD, et al. Validation of PROMIS® Physical Function computerized adaptive tests for orthopaedic foot and ankle outcome research. Clin Orthop Relat Res 2013;471(11):3466–74.

Charcot-Marie-Tooth Disease: A Surgical Algorithm

Glenn B. Pfeffer, MD*, Max P. Michalski, MD, MSc

KEYWORDS

- Cavovarus • Charcot-Marie-Tooth • Osteotomies • Soft tissue release
- Tendon transfer

KEY POINTS

- Surgical treatment of neurologic cavovarus should create a plantigrade foot, provide ankle stability with control of the hindfoot, and restore active ankle dorsiflexion.
- Precise motor testing of each muscle that controls the foot and ankle is essential.
- The surgical algorithm is dynamic and changes based on intraoperative findings after soft tissue releases.
- The need for specific osteotomies can only be determined after all necessary soft tissue releases are complete.
- The center of rotation of angulation is in the midfoot and requires an adequate release of the medial soft tissues to correct the deformity.

If you don't know where you're going, you'll end up somewhere else.

– Yogi Berra

INTRODUCTION

The cavovarus caused by Charcot-Marie-Tooth (CMT) disease often involves extreme muscle imbalance and severe deformity. Patients often seek treatment, only to be told there is nothing to do. Braces are typically considered the only option. Given the progressive nature of the disease, many wonder if there is any point in going through an operation. The surgical treatment can be daunting, and result in a suboptimal result with persistent deformity. The goal of this article is to present a multifactorial treatment algorithm that we believe will help achieve improved results. Our recommendations are based on over 700 CMT surgeries performed by the senior author over 35 years of practice.

The most common cause of a neurologic cavovarus foot is CMT disease, a hereditary motor sensory neuropathy that affects 1 in 2500 persons.[1,2] Although genetic in origin,

Department of Orthopaedic Surgery, Cedars-Sinai Medical Center, 444 South San Vicente Boulevard, Suite 603, Los Angeles, CA 90048, USA
* Corresponding author.
E-mail address: Glenn.Pfeffer@cshs.org

Foot Ankle Clin N Am 28 (2023) 857–871
https://doi.org/10.1016/j.fcl.2023.05.005
1083-7515/23/© 2023 Elsevier Inc. All rights reserved.

foot.theclinics.com

symptoms and foot deformity may not manifest until adolescence, or even adulthood. Most patients presenting to an orthopedic clinic complain of difficulty walking, foot drop, ankle instability, painful calluses, and lateral foot overload. The typical deformity involves an elevated arche, hindfoot varus, midfoot adduction, forefoot valgus, and clawed toes (**Fig. 1**). These deformities are likely secondary to muscular imbalances with the posterior tibial (PT) and peroneus longus (PL) muscles overpowering the weakened peroneus brevis (PB) and tibialis anterior (TA), in addition to intrinsic muscular wasting.[3,4] CMT is considered a length dependent neuropathy, although there are exceptions, especially in those with the axonal forms of the disease.[5] Patients with flaccid paralysis rarely require surgery as the deformity is mild without muscular imbalances, and treatment with a ground reaction ankle-foot orthosis is the best option.

Surgical planning for a CMT cavovarus reconstruction relies on both preoperative and intraoperative evaluation. An algorithmic approach is necessary, as the surgical strategy often changes throughout the operation. The next surgical procedure is often dependent on the result of the previous. Surgical treatment should focus on the 3 salient goals of neurologic cavovarus surgery: the creation of a plantigrade foot, hindfoot stability, and active ankle dorsiflexion.

PREOPERATIVE EVALUATION

Many patients have learned to live with their deformity. Impairment has become their new normal. It is important for both you and the patient to understand the limitations

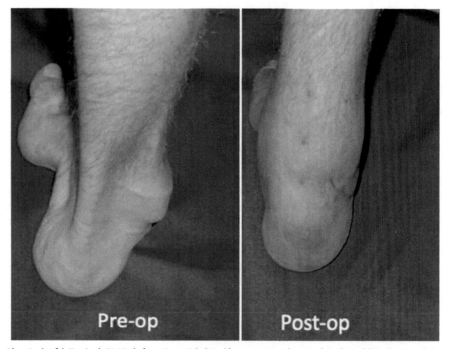

Fig. 1. (Left) Typical CMT deformity with hindfoot varus, elevated arch, adduction, and supination of the midfoot and forefoot valgus. (Right) Postoperative plantigrade positioning after medial soft tissue release, tendoachilles lengthening, calcaneal osteotomy, peroneus longus to brevis transfer, posterior tibial tendon transfer to the dorsum of the foot, and dorsal closing wedge osteotomy of the first metatarsal.

caused by the CMT. Are the toes catching on the ground from weak ankle dorsiflexion, is the ankle giving way, are there painful calluses from a nonplantigrade foot? The age of onset is important, as the longer the deformity has been present, the harder it will be to correct. Tendons and joints become increasingly contracted, and an ankle with chronic lateral laxity can become arthritic and irreducible. Deformity often progresses rapidly during adolescence, and it may be best to defer surgery for several years to follow the evolution, provided the foot remains passively reducible to a neutral position in a brace. When a foot remains "crooked" in a brace, regardless of the age of the patient, surgery is indicated. Genetic testing can be helpful, as the demyelinating CMT1A often has a more predictable presentation than the axonal forms of the disease.[6,7] Always document previous surgery done elsewhere.

PHYSICAL EXAMINATION

The physical examination can be very difficult. Patients have learned to compensate for their deformity and individual pattern of muscle weakness. The degree of their pathology may not be immediately obvious, and no 2 cases are the same. Most patients have the classic presentation of a weak PB and TA, with a strong PL and PT, but many surgeries will fail if you assume that is always the case.

Inspection

- Prior incisions, deformity, calluses, or ulceration.
- Gait–evaluate recruitment of the long toe extensors. They are often used to compensate for a weak TA and contribute to worsening of claw toe deformity.

Palpation

Tenderness may be present over plantar calluses but are often not symptomatic because of sensory neuropathy.

Range of motion (ROM)

Frequently difficult to assess because of underlying soft tissue contractures.

- Ankle joint–dorsiflexion limited.
  - Achilles contracture versus gastrocnemius contracture.
  - Tibiotalar impingement due to horizontal position of the talus and plantarflexion of the metatarsals (tibio-pedal equinus).
- Subtalar joint—passive evaluation of the ability to correct hindfoot varus.
- Talonavicular joint—passive evaluation of the ability to correct midfoot adduction.
- Metatarsal-phalangeal, PIP, and IP of great toe—Can they be passively reduced?

Strength

Most important part of the examination—check and re-check.

- Evaluate and record all muscles of the lower leg, crucial for intraop decision making (**Table 1**).
- Patients with CMT rarely have normal muscle strength; but even a weakened muscle can be used for a tendon transfer, especially if it is causing deformity.

Sensory

Often diminished, but usually not a pertinent issue in surgical planning.

Table 1	
Preoperative motor examination checklist	
Tibialis anterior	Gastro-Soleus
Extensor hallucis longus (EHL)	Posterior tibialis (PT)
Extensor digitorum longus (EDL)	Flexor hallucis longus (FHL)
Peroneus brevis (PB)	Flexor digitorum longus (FDL)
Peroneus longus (PL)	

SPECIAL TESTS

- Ankle laxity—differentiate from gait instability, which can be multifactorial (weakness, deformity, sensory abnormality).
- Coleman block—not used, except as a teaching tool. The results of this test can be confusing, as the ability to adequately reduce hindfoot varus is an intraop decision, only after soft tissue releases.[8]

The final component of the preoperative assessment is imaging, which can be difficult to interpret depending on the degree of deformity. Our typical assessment involves.

- Weight-bearing AP, oblique, and lateral views of the foot and ankle (**Fig. 2**)

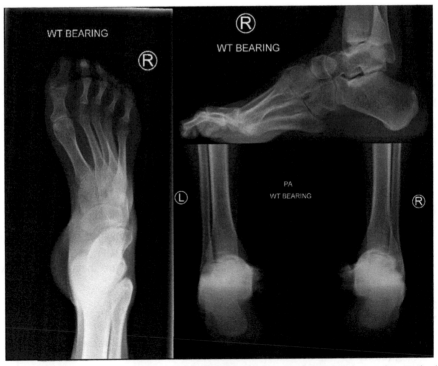

Fig. 2. (Left) AP foot radiograph demonstrating talonavicular over-coverage, talus stacked on top of the calcaneus, increased axial talo-first metatarsal angle and adduction of the forefoot. (Right superior) Lateral foot with metatarsal stacking, en face view of the subtalar posterior facet and increased sagittal talo-first metatarsal angle. (Right inferior) Saltzman view with bilateral varus hindfoot alignment angle, R > L.

- Hindfoot alignment view
- Weight-bearing CT with 3D reformats (**Fig. 3**)

With cavovarus, the metatarsals are stacked, the navicular and cuboid overlap is diminished, and the sinus tarsi is open. The supination deformity makes it frequently impossible to obtain a lateral radiograph of the foot and the ankle on the same film. Meary's angle, calcaneal pitch, ankle laxity, degenerative changes, and open growth plates should all be evaluated. The weight bearing cat scan (WBCT) 3D reformats are scrutinized to evaluate the center of the deformity (typically the TN joint), degenerative changes, and morphology of the calcaneus, which often has a smaller radius of curvature than normal.[9] A stress radiograph of the ankle is needed at some point prior to the start of surgery. It is not uncommon to see an isolated laxity of the CFL with a normal anterior talo fibular ligament (ATFL), due to the trajectory of the deformity.[10]

OPERATIVE APPROACH

The surgery can be done as an outpatient. A regional block is used for immediate post-operative pain control, and a peripheral nerve catheter has been shown to be safe and may provide up to 5 days of pain relief.[11]

Restoration of a Plantigrade Foot

The most important goal of surgery is restoration of a plantigrade foot. If nothing else, the plantigrade foot will be braceable, without abnormal loading of joints and inevitable degenerative changes. Although a triple arthrodesis can almost always achieve a plantigrade foot, a joint sparing approach is preferred to maintain motion, especially in a young patient, and is supported by prior literature indicating better long-term outcomes.[12–14] Multiple combinations of soft tissue releases, tendon transfers, and osteotomies have been described in the literature.[4,15–19]

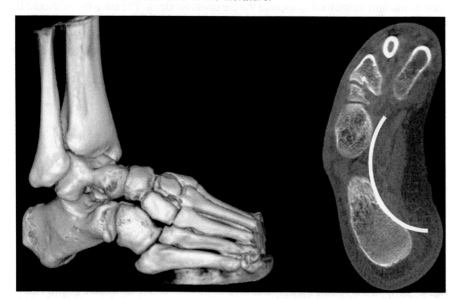

Fig. 3. (Left) 3D reformat demonstrating the center of rotation of angulation (CORA) at the talonavicular and calcaneocuboid joints. (Right) Axial evaluation of the calcaneus demonstrating a small radius of curvature ("C shaped") posterior tuberosity associated with axial varus of the heel.

In most patients, our first procedure is a triple-cut Achilles tendon lengthening. The Achilles inserts medial to the midline on the posterior tuberosity of the calcaneus. It becomes contracted as ankle dorsiflexion weakens and a foot drop develops. The contracture contributes to the varus deformity of the heel. The gastrocnemius is rarely the isolated source of the contracture. The triple-cut lengthening is done leaving the lateral insertion of the Achilles intact.

We next approach the midfoot, as most patients require a transfer of the posterior tibial tendon to the dorsum of the foot. The talonavicular joint is the site of maximal adduction (supination) in patients with CMT.[20,21] A medial release is essential to restore a plantigrade foot and involves release of the medial and dorsal talonavicular joint, spring ligament, and posterior tibial tendon (**Fig. 4**). The posterior tibial tendon is released first (see below in the section on Drop Foot). If planning a transfer of the flexor digitorum longus (FDL) or flexor hallucis longus (FHL) tendons, the tendons should be harvested through this medial incision, extended distally to obtain adequate tendon length. Very few patients require release of the medial subtalar joint. Use caution, as release of the medial subtalar ligaments can lead to overcorrection and excessive heel valgus postoperatively (**Fig. 5**). The release of these ligaments may be helpful if a subtalar fusion is planned. If the talonavicular joint remains irreducible following the soft tissue releases, a talonavicular or double fusion may be needed facilitate adequate alignment.

The next step is addressing hindfoot varus. Preoperatively it is difficult to understand which patient will require a calcaneal osteotomy, as the soft tissues have not been released. Recent literature has shown abnormal hindfoot bony morphology with a smaller radius of curvature in patients with CMT, meaning the axial plane of the calcaneus is "C" shaped. There are therefore both coronal (as viewed from posterior) and axial (as viewed from superior) components to hindfoot varus.[9]

An oblique lateral incision is made over the calcaneal tuberosity and extended to the base of the fifth metatarsal to expose the peroneal tendons. The sural nerve should be protected. This incision may be translated superior as needed to expose the peroneal tendons, and address lateral ligament instability, if needed. Multiple lateralizing osteotomies have been described including simple translational, closing wedge, and more

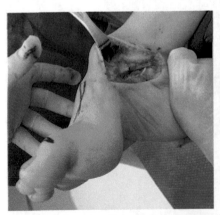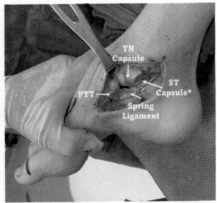

Fig. 4. (Left) medial release incision in cavovarus position before correction. (Right) Passive reduction of the foot after medial release of the dorsal and lateral talonavicular capsule, spring ligament, and posterior tibial tendon with a wafer of the navicular tuberosity. The medial subtalar joint has been released in this patient but can lead to overcorrection especially in adolescent patients. Note the plantarflexion of the first ray after correction at the midfoot.

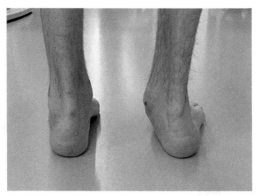

Fig. 5. Postoperative right foot following medial release that included the subtalar joint resulting in over correction and valgus deformity that required a subtalar fusion.

complex multi-dimensional osteotomies. Preoperative assessment of the calcaneus 3D reconstructions and axial bone series can provide valuable insight regarding the need for a simple lateral translation or a multi-dimensional osteotomy. In more significant deformity with a "C" shaped calcaneus, a closing wedge osteotomy in conjunction with lateral translation and coronal rotation are typically needed to correct both the axial and coronal components of the varus (**Fig. 6**).[22–24] These combined osteotomies are very powerful, and care should be taken to avoid overcorrection.

To maximize the correction through the osteotomy, it is often necessary to release through the same lateral incision the soft tissues above and below the osteotomy, including a plantar fascia release with a Steindler stripping of the intrinsic muscles. A laminar spreader distracted in the osteotomy site can also help facilitate soft tissue relaxation (**Fig. 7**). Some surgeons prefer a Z-type osteotomy in the calcaneus but it is more difficult to perform and requires a much larger incision. A percutaneous calcaneal osteotomy may suffice if there is only moderate deformity.

The final step in restoration of a plantigrade foot is forefoot balancing. In the majority of patients, as the supination of the midfoot is corrected, the valgus of the forefoot increases (see **Fig. 4**, right). The first ray becomes further plantarflexed. The rotation typically occurs around the axis of the second ray. This correction is typically the penultimate step of the procedure prior to docking tendon transfers into the bone. A dorsal closing wedge osteotomy of the proximal first metatarsal is the most common technique used. Even though the plantar fascia has been released proximally, an additional release in the midfoot is often needed with significant deformity to allow dorsiflexion of the first ray. Although not intuitive, releasing the plantar fascia in the midfoot after prior release in the hindfoot typically allows additional dorsiflexion of the first ray. The goal of correction is to elevate the first metatarsal to a point level with the second. An additional closing wedge can be performed on the second metatarsal as needed. In patients with an open first metatarsal growth plate, we typically perform an opening wedge osteotomy of the medial cuneiform with an allograft.[25] A Cole osteotomy through the midfoot is indicated if more than the first and second rays are plantarflexed.[26] In our experience, a Cole osteotomy is required in fewer than 5% of patients.

ANKLE STABILITY AND CONTROL OF THE HINDFOOT

Prior to prepping and draping the patient, ankle stability is checked with a fluoroscopic stress examination. This information is used to plan incisions. If unstable, the CFL is

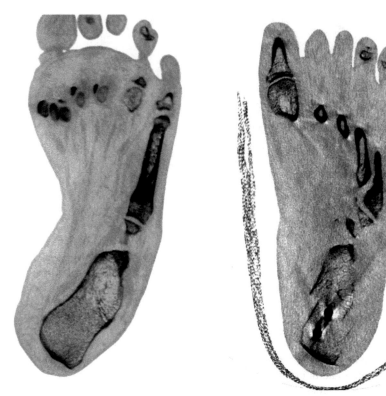

Fig. 6. Pre- and postoperative axial WBCT slices at the posterior tuberosity. Contrast has been inverted for finer anatomic detail. (Left) Preoperative image with a small radius of curvature at the posterior tuberosity of the calcaneus. (Right) Postoperative image demonstrating lateral translation and less curvature at the medial border using a lateral closing wedge.

repaired through the incision used to access the peroneal tendons, often augmented with nonabsorbable suture tape. Interestingly, in these relatively low activity patients, the ATFL is rarely lax, only the CFL (from chronic varus stress).

Control of the hindfoot is ideally restored with tendon transfers for a dynamic correction, but alternatively can be achieved through fusion. A fusion, usually of the subtalar joint, is only needed if there is no muscle of adequate strength to transfer. Most commonly, the peroneus longus is transferred to the brevis tendon with a 3 pass pulvertaft weave distal to the fibula (**Fig. 8**). The preoperative examination is crucial at this stage. If the peroneus longus has no excursion or preoperatively provides no eversion strength, alternative muscles must be used. If the FHL tendon had good power, it can be harvested through the medial incision, rerouted behind the fibula, passed distally within the peroneal tunnel, and woven into the distal peroneus brevis. If the peroneal tendons are dysfunctional, based on preoperative examination and intraoperative evaluation, they can be completely excised within the peroneal tunnel, to leave adequate room for the FHL transfer. The PB stump is typically left intact distal to the tip of the fibula to weave the transferred tendon. Rarely is the tendon transferred into the base of the fifth metatarsal, although that is an option. The flexor digitorum is an alternative tendon to transfer but has less strength than the FHL.

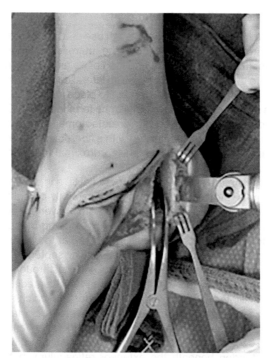

Fig. 7. Lateral incision used to address peroneals and calcaneal osteotomy. The soft tissues above and below the posterior tuberosity have been released. A laminar spreader has been inserted to stretch the soft tissues and allow for stress relaxation. The second cut of the osteotomy is posterior and oblique. This can be performed with the laminar spreader in place to visualize the exit trajectory of the posterior cut.

In more advanced disease, only the Achilles and PT have preserved strength. In these patients, an excellent option is a fusion of the subtalar or talonavicular joint, in conjunction with a transfer of the PT for active ankle dorsiflexion. Another option is a Bridle procedure[27,28]; this transfer, however, relies on an already weakened PT to provide both dorsiflexion and eversion power.

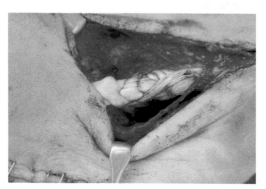

Fig. 8. Pulvertaft weave of the peroneus longus into the peroneus brevis insertion stump. The tendon has been passed through the brevis tendon 3 times and secured in maximal eversion. This patient had a dual incision approach to the peroneals and calcaneal osteotomy although both are typically addressed through a single lateral incision.

Restoration of Ankle Dorsiflexion Strength

Most commonly, dorsiflexion is restored through use of a posterior tibial tendon transfer, redirected posterior to the tibia, through the interosseous membrane, down the anterior compartment between the tibia and the tibialis anterior, beneath the extensor retinaculum and into the lateral cuneiform.[29] The lateral cuneiform is the central axis of the foot. Obtaining enough length of the tendon to place into the cuneiform is key. The tendon should be dissected out to its medial cuneiform insertion. Often a small wafer of the medial navicular has to be raised with an osteotome to preserve adequate thickness in the tendon, which is then tubularized with a fiber-loop suture (**Fig. 9**).[30] Usually, the posterior tibial sheath needs to be released proximal to the medial malleolus to pass the distal stump proximally.

A second incision is made along the posteromedial tibia in the distal third of the leg. The flexor digitorum is retraced aside and the PT carefully brought into the proximal incision. A third incision is made just lateral to the tibia, over the tibialis anterior. The incision should be distal to the medial incision, overlapping by approximately 50%. The neurovascular bundle must be carefully protected at the base of the lateral incision. A small freer is used to pierce the intermuscular septum several times at the base of the lateral incision. This makes creation of a tunnel through the septum easier. A large peon clamp is passed through the septum from the medial incision. It is then widely spread to facilitate tendon passage and excursion which should be approximately 5 cm.[31] An additional peon clamp is then passed from lateral to medial, as the medial clamp is withdrawn by clamping them together. The tendon is then passed by withdrawing the second peon back through the lateral incision with the tendon. We typically pass the tendon beneath the extensor retinaculum, but if more length is needed to reach the lateral cuneiform, it can be redirected subcutaneously with the peon clamp, which creates a more direct course of the transfer.[32] The tendon is measured, and an appropriate drill hole is made in the lateral cuneiform, through a separate incision on the foot. The tendon is passed with a beath pin, directed to avoid the plantar neurovascular bundle. Fixation of this tendon is the final step before closure. During this step, the tendon excursion is checked with the ankle held in neutral. Final tension is approximately 75% of maximal tension (dorsiflexion) but never maximal tension as this can cause a calcaneus gait. The biotenodesis screw is typically inserted a few turns to hold then tendon and the excursion is checked. The screw is often withdrawn, and this is repeated until optimal tension is set and then the screw fully advanced into the tunnel.

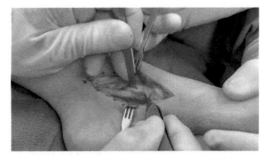

Fig. 9. Posterior tibial tendon harvest. An osteotome is used to take a wafer of bone with the navicular insertion of the posterior tibial tendon to allow tendon dissection distally to the insertions under the cuneiforms and maximize length for transfer.

In cases where the preoperative examination showed suboptimal strength of the posterior tibial tendon, we will augment the transfer with the FDL, if functioning, which is passed alongside the posterior tibial tendon, and transferred into the medial cuneiform and the posterior tibial tendon into the lateral cuneiform. Alternatively, patients who have preserved strength in the long toe extensors, the extensor hallucis longus (EHL) and extensor digitorum longus (EDL) can be transferred into either the cuneiforms or metatarsals which has been demonstrated to increase their dorsiflexion power, while eliminating their deforming force on the toes (**Fig. 10**).[33] The EHL is typically transferred into the medial cuneiform and the EDL into the lateral cuneiform. In this case, the interphalangeal joint (IP) of the great toe and proximal interphalangeal joints (PIP) of the lesser toes should usually be fused to prevent a progressive flexion deformity postoperatively. These patients typically have narrowed phalangeal bones that are too small for an implant and may only accept a 0.045″ k wire which is left for 2 weeks. Percutaneous tenotomies of the lesser toes should also be considered.

Charcot-Marie-Tooth cavovarus reconstruction algorithm
Position: Supine with large bump under the ipsilateral hip, as long as hip motion is adequate to rotate the leg for medial exposure.

Procedure
- Stress fluoroscopic examination—varus and anterior drawer.
  - If abnormal, address through peroneal/calcaneal osteotomy incision.
  - Typically only the calcaneal fibular ligament (CFL) is repaired by excising redundant tissue and augmented with a suture tape construct.

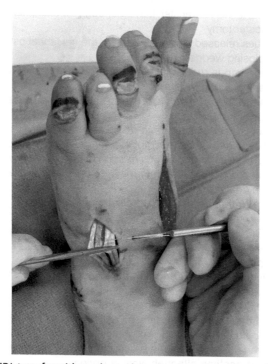

Fig. 10. EHL and EDL transfer with tendons released and anchored through midfoot incision. IP/PIP have been exposed for fusion to prevent further clawing after removal of the long extensors. This is frequently a staged procedure after the primary cavovarus reconstruction.

- Talonavicular (TAL)—triple cut with #11 blade, leave the distal stump inserted laterally for valgus pull.
- Medial release—along the course of the PT, extended to medial cuneiform. Identify and protect the TA.
  - Dorsal and medial TN capsule, spring ligament and PT harvest.
    - Rarely release subtalar joint as well but can be performed in severe deformity, beware of overcorrection.
  - Incision extended distally if FDL or FHL transfers needed to augment dorsiflexion or eversion.
    - Abductor fascia may be contracted and released through this incision.
  - PT is pulled proximally and then through IOM into the anterior compartment, and it is left until later in the case, to prevent desiccation.
  - If unable to reduce the TN joint despite adequate release, opt for a talonavicular fusion with enough bony resection for adequate correction. A TN and subtalar fusion may be required in this case.
- Lateral incision—oblique over the posterior tuberosity of the calcaneus extended to the base of the 5th. Provides access for calcaneal osteotomy, peroneals, and lateral ligament repair if necessary.
  - Peroneals
    - Peroneus longus released distally below the cuboid. This is performed even if no function to facilitate correction of forefoot valgus.
      - Assess for excursion. If none or no preoperative strength, will plan for FHL or FDL transfer into the brevis, or fusion of either TN ± ST joint.
    - If both peroneals are dysfunctional, they are excised to make more room in the peroneal tunnel for transfer, leaving enough PB stump for a Pulvertaft weave.
  - Calcaneal osteotomy
    - Soft tissues released above and below the calcaneal osteotomy site.
    - Lateral closing wedge osteotomy.
      - Anterior limb is medial to lateral and posterior cut is oblique to prevent shortening with translation.
      - 5–8 mm wedge corrects axial varus and decompresses hindfoot allowing tuberosity translation.
      - Laminar spreader inserted to distract and allow stress relaxation.
      - PF release and Steindler stripping of the intrinsic muscles
      - Lateral translation and valgus rotation of the posterior tuberosity added to the osteotomy in severe deformity. Be cautious for overcorrection, especially in adolescents.
      - Fixation with 2 antegrade partially threaded screws
  - Lateral ligaments
    - Repair CF ± ATFL depending on preop stress fluoroscopy examination. Typically only CFL required.
  - Return to peroneals
    - Typically transfer the PL through the insertion of the PB tendon with a pulvertaft weave using 3 passes.
      - Typically tensioned in maximal eversion that acts to stabilize the hindfoot even if the if disease progresses and PL loses strength.
    - If PL is nonfunctional or lacks excursion, pass the FHL posterior to the fibula and pulvertaft weave into the brevis stump with similar tension in eversion. The FDL is another, although weaker option.
    - Alternative would be a subtalar or talonavicular fusion if no viable tendon available for transfer.

- Forefoot—assess position of the first ray. There is typically worsened plantarflexion deformity after correction of midfoot and hindfoot deformities.
  ○ Secondary PF release in the midfoot through a small plantar incision. The first ray may completely correct with PF and PL releases.
  ○ If remains plantarflexed, dorsal first metatarsal incision for osteotomy.
    ▪ Dorsal closing wedge in the proximal metatarsal, fixation with a single screw in the proximal segment, and tension band wire passed through the distal segment.
      • Elevate to level of second metatarsal.
    ▪ Similar procedure can be done to the second metatarsal and leveled with the rest of the metatarsal heads.
  ○ Open growth plate—perform osteotomy in the cuneiform. An opening wedge with an allograft will also abduct the ray that is usually desirable.
  ○ Plantarflexion of entire forefoot can be corrected with a Cole midfoot osteotomy performed through the medial release and long lateral incisions.
- Restoration of active ankle dorsiflexion—dorsal midfoot incision localized with fluoroscopy over lateral cuneiform.
  ○ Tendon transfer fixation performed last before closure.
  ○ Post tib ± FDL inserted into the lateral (± medial) cuneiform with biotenodesis screw, tensioned 25% short of maximal dorsiflexion excursion. Err on the side of too tight than loose but not in maximal tension.
  ○ If transferring EHL or EDL, harvest tendons in the midfoot and transfer into the cuneiforms (proximal metatarsals are an alternative option).
    ▪ Fuse IP/PIP joints if transferring EHL ± EDL tendons as a flexion deformity through the joints will often occur.
    ▪ Percutaneous flexor tenotomies, if needed to balance the toes.

Postoperative Protocol

The surgery is typically performed as an outpatient with regional nerve catheters utilized for adjunctive pain control. Sterile dressings and a well-padded plaster short leg splint are placed at the culmination of the procedure. The patient is immobilized and nonweight bearing on the surgical limb for 6 weeks postoperatively. The splint is changed at 2 weeks postoperatively where wounds are assessed, and sutures are likely removed. The patient is transitioned to a fiberglass short leg cast to complete the period of immobilization and nonweight bearing. At week 6 postoperatively, the patient may begin weight bearing while utilizing a CAM walker boot which is only removed for hygiene. Physical therapy referral is initiated at 8 weeks to begin active range-of-motion exercises and begin gait training out of the boot. At this point, the patient may progress to regular tennis shoes, and begin to resume activities at their own tolerance.

COMPLICATIONS

Complications associated with cavovarus reconstructions include wound breakdown given the numerous incisions, overcorrection especially when releasing the subtalar joint in adolescents, recurrent ankle instability, and symptomatic hardware. Additionally, unique to neurologic cavovarus surgery, the disease and muscle weakness may progress and require future bracing or repeat surgery.

SUMMARY

A regimented approach is critical to create a plantigrade foot, restore hindfoot stability, and generate active ankle dorsiflexion. The preoperative motor examination is fundamental to the algorithm as it is the cornerstone of surgical planning. Surgeons need to be comfortable with multiple techniques to achieve each surgical goal. Each patient with CMT presents differently, with varying degrees of muscle imbalance, soft tissue contractures, and deformity. A plantigrade foot is the most important of the surgical goals as hindfoot stability and ankle dorsiflexion can be augmented with bracing. Soft tissues must be released before osteotomies are considered.

DISCLOSURES

The authors have nothing to disclose.

REFERENCES

1. Laura M, Singh D, Ramdharry G, et al. Prevalence and orthopedic management of foot and ankle deformities in Charcot-Marie-Tooth disease. Muscle Nerve 2018; 57(2):255–9.
2. Martyn CN, Hughes RA. Epidemiology of peripheral neuropathy. J Neurol Neurosurg Psychiatr 1997;62(4):310–8.
3. Aminian A, Sangeorzan BJ. The anatomy of cavus foot deformity. Foot Ankle Clin 2008;13(2):191–8, v.
4. Beals TC, Nickisch F. Charcot-marie-tooth disease and the cavovarus foot. Foot Ankle Clin 2008;13(2):259–74, vi-vii.
5. Patzko A, Shy ME. Update on charcot-marie-tooth disease. Curr Neurol Neurosci Rep 2011;11(1):78–88.
6. Gemelli C, Geroldi A, Massucco S, et al. Genetic workup for charcot-marie-tooth neuropathy: a retrospective single-site experience covering 15 years. Life 2022; 12(3):402.
7. Panosyan FB, Laura M, Rossor AM, et al. Cross-sectional analysis of a large cohort with X-linked Charcot-Marie-Tooth disease (CMTX1). Neurology 2017; 89(9):927–35.
8. Pfeffer GB, Gonzalez T, Brodsky J, et al. A consensus statement on the surgical treatment of charcot-marie-tooth disease. Foot Ankle Int 2020;41(7):870–80.
9. Michalski MP, An TW, Haupt ET, et al. Abnormal bone morphology in charcot-marie-tooth disease. Foot Ankle Int 2022;43(4):576–81.
10. Waldman LE, Michalski MP, Giaconi JC, et al. Charcot-marie-tooth disease of the foot and ankle: imaging features and pathophysiology. Radiographics 2023; 43(4):e220114.
11. An T, Schwartz E, Kissen M, et al. Safety and efficacy of postoperative indwelling popliteal nerve catheters for outpatient charcot-marie-tooth surgery. Foot Ankle Int 2022;43(4):504–8.
12. Tejero S, Chans-Veres J, Carranza-Bencano A, et al. Functional results and quality of life after joint preserving or sacrificing surgery in Charcot-Marie-Tooth foot deformities. Int Orthop 2021;45(10):2569–78.
13. Ward CM, Dolan LA, Bennett DL, et al. Long-term results of reconstruction for treatment of a flexible cavovarus foot in Charcot-Marie-Tooth disease. J Bone Joint Surg Am 2008;90(12):2631–42.
14. Wetmore RS, Drennan JC. Long-term results of triple arthrodesis in Charcot-Marie-Tooth disease. J Bone Joint Surg Am 1989;71(3):417–22.
15. Leeuwesteijn AE, de Visser E, Louwerens JW. Flexible cavovarus feet in Charcot-Marie-Tooth disease treated with first ray proximal dorsiflexion osteotomy combined with soft tissue surgery: a short-term to mid-term outcome study. Foot Ankle Surg 2010;16(3):142–7.

16. Sammarco GJ. Osteotomy of the foot and ankle. Foot Ankle Clin 2001;6(3):xi–xiii.
17. Sammarco GJ, Taylor R. Combined calcaneal and metatarsal osteotomies for the treatment of cavus foot. Foot Ankle Clin 2001;6(3):533–43, vii.
18. Wicart P, Seringe R. Plantar opening-wedge osteotomy of cuneiform bones combined with selective plantar release and dwyer osteotomy for pes cavovarus in children. J Pediatr Orthop 2006;26(1):100–8.
19. Togei K, Shima H, Tsujinaka S, et al. Joint preserving procedures for painful plantar callosities in patients with flexible cavovarus foot. Foot Ankle Surg 2022;28(7):1094–9.
20. An T, Haupt E, Michalski M, et al. Cavovarus with a twist: midfoot coronal and axial plane rotational deformity in charcot-marie-tooth disease. Foot Ankle Int 2022;43(5):676–82.
21. Ranjit S, Sangoi D, Cullen N, et al. Assessing the coronal plane deformity in Charcot Marie Tooth Cavovarus feet using automated 3D measurements. Foot Ankle Surg 2023. https://doi.org/10.1016/j.fas.2023.02.013.
22. An TW, Michalski M, Jansson K, et al. Comparison of lateralizing calcaneal osteotomies for varus hindfoot correction. Foot Ankle Int 2018;39(10):1229–36.
23. Cody EA, Kraszewski AP, Conti MS, et al. Lateralizing calcaneal osteotomies and their effect on calcaneal alignment: a three-dimensional digital model analysis. Foot Ankle Int 2018;39(8):970–7.
24. Pfeffer GB, Michalski MP, Basak T, et al. Use of 3D prints to compare the efficacy of three different calcaneal osteotomies for the correction of heel varus. Foot Ankle Int 2018;39(5):591–7.
25. Mosca VS. The cavus foot. J Pediatr Orthop 2001;21(4):423–4.
26. Cole WH. The treatment of claw-foot. Clin Orthop Relat Res 1983;(181):3–6.
27. Johnson JE, Paxton ES, Lippe J, et al. Outcomes of the bridle procedure for the treatment of foot drop. Foot Ankle Int 2015;36(11):1287–96.
28. Rodriguez RP. The Bridle procedure in the treatment of paralysis of the foot. Foot Ankle 1992;13(2):63–9.
29. Dreher T, Wolf SI, Heitzmann D, et al. Tibialis posterior tendon transfer corrects the foot drop component of cavovarus foot deformity in Charcot-Marie-Tooth disease. J Bone Joint Surg Am 2014;96(6):456–62.
30. Haupt ET, Chan JY, Michalski M, et al. Evaluation and management of adult footdrop. J Am Acad Orthop Surg 2022;30(16):747–56.
31. Wagner P, Ortiz C, Vela O, et al. Interosseous membrane window size for tibialis posterior tendon transfer-Geometrical and MRI analysis. Foot Ankle Surg 2016; 22(3):196–9.
32. Wagner E, Wagner P, Zanolli D, et al. Biomechanical evaluation of circumtibial and transmembranous routes for posterior tibial tendon transfer for dropfoot. Foot Ankle Int 2018;39(7):843–9.
33. Pfeffer GB, Michalski M, Nelson T, et al. Extensor tendon transfers for treatment of foot drop in charcot-marie-tooth disease: a biomechanical evaluation. Foot Ankle Int 2020;41(4):449–56.

Managing Cavovarus Feet in Diabetic Patients

Madhu Tiruveedhula, FRCSGlasg(Orth)[a],*,
Venu Kavarthapu, FRCS(Orth)[b]

KEYWORDS

- Cavovarus foot • Diabetic peripheral neuropathy • Coleman block test
- Charcot neuroarthropathy

KEY POINTS

- Cavovarus foot deformity can be of familial non-neurologic cause or associated with an underlying neurologic condition, the most common being the Charcot–Marie–Tooth disease.
- Diabetic motor neuropathy can lead to a cavovarus foot from resultant soft tissue imbalances and contracture of muscle and tendons.
- In patients with insensate feet, the calluses under the bony prominences break down to ulceration very early in the disease; hence, nonoperative treatment has a high risk of failure.
- There is paucity of published guidelines on the management of diabetic peripheral neuropathy exacerbated cavovarus feet; hence, three stages of the disease and their treatment strategy are described.

INTRODUCTION

A cavovarus foot is characterized by exacerbated medial longitudinal arch (cavus), hindfoot varus, plantar-flexed first ray, forefoot protonation (apparent supination), forefoot adduction, and claw toe deformities.[1] It can be broadly divided as flexible and rigid, with a flexible deformity seen in younger patients gradually progressing to fixed deformities.[2]

This can be further classified by the cause of the deformity. The most common being the idiopathic subtle cavovarus feet with mild hindfoot varus and plantar-flexed first ray. The familial non-neurologic cause is the next common and is associated with cavovarus feet with all the features described but with no obvious muscle weakness. The neurologic cavovarus feet is characterized by weakness of peroneal brevis, tibialis anterior muscle and intrinsic muscles of the toes with compensatory overpowering

[a] Mid & South Essex Foundation NHS Trust, Basildon Hospital, Nethermayne, Basildon SS16 5NL, UK; [b] King's College Hospital, Denmark Hill, London, SE5 9RS, UK
* Corresponding author.
E-mail address: madhutiruveedhula@gmail.com

Foot Ankle Clin N Am 28 (2023) 873–887
https://doi.org/10.1016/j.fcl.2023.05.006   foot.theclinics.com

of peroneal longus, tibialis posterior, gastroc-soleus muscle complex, and plantar aponeurosis.[3]

The neurologic cavovarus foot can be further divided as progressive and nonprogressive; Charcot–Marie–Tooth disease (CMT), a form of hereditary sensory motor neuropathy is the most common progressive neurologic cause, seen in 100 individuals per million.[3,4] The other causes being the conditions that affect the central nervous system such as strokes, Friedreich's ataxia, spinal causes such as tethered cord or a spinal cord tumor, and traumatic cause such as sequelae of compartment syndrome. Peripheral neuropathy from diabetes is associated with a cavovarus deformity as well.[5] The nonprogressive form is seen in patients with cerebral palsy, poliomyelitis, or with myelomeningocele.[4]

Patients with CMT are characterized by distal extremity weakness with foot muscles supplied by the tibial nerve are affected first.[4] The clinical signs characteristic of CMT are plantar-flexed first ray from overpowering of peroneal longus muscle, progressive hindfoot varus and apparent midfoot supination (true protonation) and adduction from tightness of tibialis posterior muscle, and progressive claw toe deformity of all toes from intrinsic muscle wasting and hypertrophy of plantar fascia.[6] The dorsiflexion deformities of the toes worsen the windlass mechanism exacerbating the tightness of plantar fascia resulting in its tears. The deformity is flexible to start with but becomes rigid rapidly in patients with neurologic causes.[2,3,7]

The Coleman block test is a helpful clinical diagnostic tool to differentiate if the hindfoot varus is a flexible forefoot-driven deformity or a fixed deformity.[8] When standing on a 1-inch block, with the lateral column of the foot on the block, patient is asked to drop the first ray of the foot. If the hindfoot varus corrects to 5° of valgus, then the cavovarus deformity is a forefoot-driven one, from the overpowering of the peroneal longus muscle.[7,8]

Diabetes and Cavovarus Feet

Diabetes commonly results in a flat foot from rocker-bottom deformity due to Charcot neuroarthropathy (CN). However, diabetic peripheral neuropathy with a marked motor component affecting the muscles of foot and ankle can result in a cavovarus deformity due to muscle imbalance and exacerbated muscle/tendon contractures. The associated loss of protective sensation from neuropathy and autonomic dysfunction contribute to focal callosities at bony prominences very early, which break down to ulceration.[5]

Diabetes-induced increased glycosylation of type 1 collagen fibers results in short and stiff muscle-tendon complexes.[9] This exacerbates the stronger muscles seen in patients with neurologic cavovarus feet such as the tibialis posterior mainly and also the peroneal longus, plantar fascia, and gastroc-soleus muscle groups. This results in progressive worsening of cavovarus deformity such as the hindfoot varus which becomes stiff rapidly progressing on to the ankle CN from collapse of medial body of talus. plantar-flexed first ray, claw toe deformities, and callus/ulceration under the middle metatarsal heads. Other associated factors such as previous surgical debridement of infected ulcers resulting in bone and soft tissue loss and prolonged immobilization in a total contact cast (TCC) can exacerbate these deformities and rigidity of the joints. Inadvertent lateral ray amputation for an ulcer or osteomyelitis, without restoring the function of peroneus brevis, can further exacerbate the midfoot deformity in patients with cavovarus foot. The location of ulceration and progression can vary markedly due to these additional factors when compared with patients with CMT without diabetes-induced peripheral neuropathy.

Based on the location and flexibility of the deformity, the focal plantar pressures progressively worsen under the bone prominences resulting in calluses which can breakdown to ulceration from increased shear stress with unprotected walking.[10] Rigid hindfoot varus and midfoot apparent supination results in calluses under the plantar surface of the base of fifth metatarsal/cuboid and under the fifth metatarsal head (**Fig. 1**). Progressive worsening of fixed hindfoot varus results in ankle CN from lateral instability due to attenuation of lateral ligament structures and progressive collapse of the medial body of talus (**Fig. 2**). This can lead to ulceration under the prominent lateral malleolus with unprotected weight-bearing, base of fifth metatarsal head/cuboid and neck of fifth metatarsal. Excessive forefoot adduction can further result in CN of the lateral column of the midfoot.[11] In addition, the tightness of peroneal longus can result in callosity/ulceration under the first metatarsal head and tightness of gastroc-soleus-tendo-Achilles complex can result in callus/ulceration under the middle toe metatarsal heads (**Fig. 3**).

Accommodative shoes and TCC can offload the areas of peak plantar pressures and calluses, however, as the deforming forces are not corrected, these calluses often breakdown to ulcers while in TCC or soon after the completion of cast treatment.[12]

The role of a multidisciplinary diabetic foot team (MDFT) is paramount in preoperative optimization of patients requiring surgical management. This includes correction of glycaemic status, renal and other medical associated comorbidities, and vascular

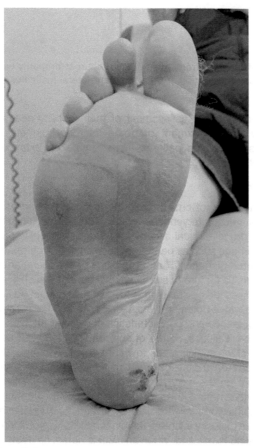

Fig. 1. Cavovarus foot deformity with callus under the cuboid and fifth metatarsal.

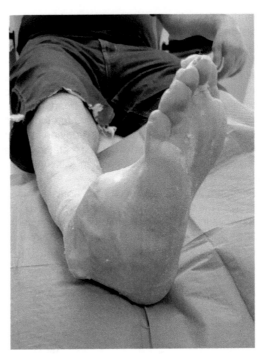

Fig. 2. Severe hindfoot varus from ankle Charcot neuroarthropathy with collapse of talus. Patient has high risk of ulceration at the prominent lateral malleolus.

assessment. In addition, the assessment of their mobility needs postsurgery, and more importantly, the adjustment of home microenvironment to adapt to non-weight bearing is critical, as patients often require an extended period of non-weight bearing after surgery.[13]

Clinical Assessment

This starts with a history of onset, location, and progression of callosity, previous nonsurgical and surgical interventions, control of diabetes, history of smoking, and other recreational drugs. Clinical assessment starts with looking for signs of associated end-organ damage such as peripheral neuropathy, nephropathy and retinopathy termed, "complicated diabetes,"[14] and presence of peripheral arterial disease.

"Peek-a-boo sign," a feature of subtle cavovarus foot, which is a medial projection of the heel when assessed on standing in front of the patient and flexibility of hindfoot varus, as assessed with a Coleman block test is noted.[7,8] The location and flexibility of foot deformities, presence and characteristics of calluses such as its thickness when compared with other calluses, nature of surrounding skin such as cellulites, hemorrhagic blister, and signs of skin breakdown are noted. For larger deformities, the examination is focused on the assessment of flexibility of joints, tibio-calcaneal and tibio-talar alignment on the axial and coronal plane, and the flexibility of the claw toes. In addition, the motor power of peroneals, tibialis anterior, tibialis posterior, gastrocnemius-soleus complex, toe intrinsics, and long toe flexors and extensors are charted. When a callosity is noted, its relation to bony prominence and likely muscle group contributing to this and, when an ulcer is noted, its depth is assessed as per the University of Texas Diabetic Wound Classification System.[15]

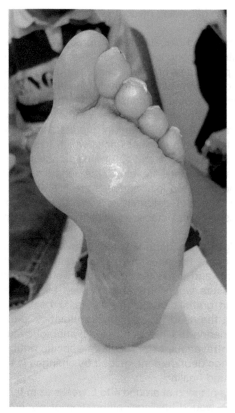

Fig. 3. Cavovarus foot with claw toe deformities with callus at the tip of the third toe and under the middle metatarsal heads suggestive of tightness of gastroc-soleus-tendo-Achilles complex + plantar flexed metatarsal head resulting in increased plantar forefoot pressures.

Standard weight-bearing radiographs of the foot and ankle are helpful to assess the degree of the deformity and to rule out associated fractures. Additional imaging includes weight-bearing computed tomography (CT) scan or standard CT scan with 3D reconstruction; this can help in planning corrective osteotomies.[11,13] In patients with an ulcer, MR imaging scan of the relevant section of the foot or ankle is indicated to assess the location and extent of osteomyelitis. A pedobarograph can provide a visual chart of the plantar pressures when standing and walking, which is valuable in patients with subtle deformities and to identify the location and degree of peak plantar pressures and useful guide for post-intervention monitoring. Vascular assessment includes digital examination of peripheral foot pulses and when in doubt, assessment of a waveform with a hand-held Doppler and arterial duplex ultrasound scan can quantify distal perfusion. Preoperative multiple soft tissue and bone biopsy samples are a valuable diagnostic tool to guide postoperative antibiotic therapy.

Management Principles

Cavovarus foot deformities that are flexible and non-ulcerated can be managed in custom orthosis or accommodative shoes but monitored closely for the deterioration of callosity to ulceration.[10,12] The earliest sign of this is change of callus to a hemorrhagic blister.[10] Severe, rigid, and progressive deformities with calluses and ulcerations often do not respond to offloading measures, and hence, early surgical correction is strongly advised.

Patients with complicated diabetes require preoperative medical optimization by the MDFT. In patients with peripheral arterial disease, vascular optimization with angioplasty or bypass procedures improves tissue perfusion, essential for wound healing. In the presence of osteomyelitis or actively infected ulcer, a staged procedure for the deformity correction should be considered.[13] The first stage of this two-stage procedure consists of surgical debridement of the ulcer, excision of devitalized bony fragments, intramedullary curettage for metatarsal osteomyelitis, multiple drill holes and irrigation for tarsal and other bones which has signs of osteomyelitis on MR imaging scan.[16] Multiple bone and soft tissue samples are obtained for microbiological analysis. The dead space created by the debridement and the curetted intramedullary canals and prepared joint surfaces are filled with local antibiotic eluting calcium preparation. The foot deformity is corrected with corrective osteotomies based on CT assessment and stabilized with threaded 3.2 mm wires or external fixator.[13]

The ulcerated edges once debrided and following corrective osteotomies, in most situations, become lax enough to close primarily without tension. When the gap is significant, and if the tension at the wound edges is likely, then the use of negative pressure wound therapy followed by delayed split skin graft or use of synthetic skin grafts can aid the ulcers to heal. After the initial broad-spectrum antibiotics, the need for additional antibiotics is planned based on the culture results considering the injection of local antibiotic eluting agents. The authors routinely use intravenous or oral culture-specific antibiotics for a minimum 2 weeks post-first stage debridement, guided by changes in the C-reactive protein (CRP) levels and wound healing.

The second stage is planned at around 4 to 6 weeks from the first stage guided by the normality of CRP, wound healing, optimization of glycemic control, and distal vascular perfusion. The choice of implants is guided by the presence of residual infection, patients' ability to cope with non-weight bearing, and the condition of soft tissues as guided by MDFT. The investigators' preferred option is to use all internal fixation method based on the principles of "durable long-segment rigid internal fixation with optimal bone opposition,"[17] the other options being external fixation with a circular frame. Before the second stage, preoperative radiographs will guide the need for additional osteotomies. Additional soft tissue and bone samples during the second stage will guide the need for postoperative antibiotics, modified as guided by CRP and wound healing. The surgical aim is to achieve a plantigrade foot with restoration of calcaneal pitch and the lateral and dorsal Meary's line.

When all internal fixation method is used, following surgery the leg is immobilized initially in a back-slab then changed to a non-weight-bearing TCC when the swelling has subsided. Patients are prescribed appropriate thromboprophylaxis based on the HAS-BLED risk assessment tool for the duration of plaster immobilization.[18] Patients are strongly advised to mobilize non-weight bearing in the TCC for a minimum 6 weeks to 3 months, modified based stability of fixation and fusion on weight-bearing radiographs and thereafter can mobilize in a brace or a surgical shoe.

Classification of Cavovarus Feet in Patients with Diabetes

The evidence from the published literature is sparse regarding a reliable guide to the management of exacerbated cavovarus deformity seen in patients with diabetic peripheral neuropathy. Guided by the literature on nondiabetic neurologic cavovarus feet and authors' own clinical experience in managing patients with such presentations, three clinical stages with their treatment strategies are described.

Stage 1: non-neurologic cavovarus feet
This stage is characterized by patients with cavovarus feet with normal power of peroneal brevis and tibialis anterior muscle group. When seen in patients with diabetic peripheral neuropathy, the deformity can progress but slowly with signs of callus and ulceration under the bony prominences secondary to sensory neuropathy.

Stage 1A: subtle cavovarus feet
This is a common, idiopathic, nonfamilial foot characterized by subtle hindfoot varus with a classic, "peek-a-boo sign."[7] The medial arch may be of normal height but has mild plantar-flexed first ray from the tightness of peroneal longus muscle and no claw toe deformities.

In patients with diabetic peripheral neuropathy and subtle cavovarus feet, callus may be seen under the first metatarsal head and possibly under the plantar surface of the fifth metatarsal/cuboid region (see **Fig. 1**). Additional callus can be seen under the middle metatarsal heads from tightness of the calf muscle complex. The deformity is flexible and these calluses unlikely to breakdown to ulceration with adequate offloading.

Stage 1B: non-neurologic rigid cavovarus feet
This is a cavovarus feet with classic deformities described above with normal power of peroneal brevis and tibialis anterior muscle groups. When complicated with diabetic peripheral neuropathy with progressive tightness of tibialis posterior muscle, the hindfoot varus progressively becomes stiff resulting in apparent midfoot supination and callosity initially and ulceration at later stages under the base of fifth metatarsal or cuboid (**Fig. 4**).

With progressive hindfoot varus, patients present with symptoms of lateral ankle instability and/or stress fractures of fifth metatarsal (**Fig. 5**). The claw toe deformities are mild and flexible in majority and rarely cause ulcerations.

Treatment Strategy

The management in these two-stages depends on the degree of flexibility of joints, passive correction of deformities, characteristic of callus and its progression to ulceration, and lastly the degree of flexibility of hindfoot varus.

In patients with Stage 1A disease, the foot is flexible, and the calluses are minor; they rarely progress to ulceration except in advanced neuropathy with marked hindfoot varus (Stage 1B). Hence, the nonoperative treatment of patients with Stage 1A disease is often accommodative shoes or custom orthosis. Regular monitoring for the progression of callus is recommended as the neuropathy progresses.

Patients with positive coleman block test
This indicates a forefoot-driven hindfoot varus, hence corrected with a combination of soft tissue procedures and selective bony osteotomies. The procedure starts with peroneal longus to peroneal brevis tenodesis behind the lateral malleolus and release of distal peroneal longus tendon ± percutaneous plantar fascial release reducing the deforming plantar flexor force on the first ray.[2,19] If the first ray remains plantar flexed but flexible, this can be corrected with Jones transfer of extensor hallucis longus tendon to the first metatarsal neck. In patients with rigid first ray or with partial correction after the soft tissue releases, a dorsal closing wedge osteotomy of the first metatarsal corrects this deformity. Once the first ray is corrected, the hindfoot tibio-calcaneal

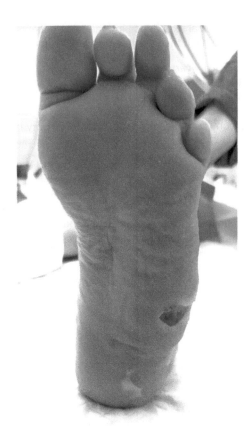

Fig. 4. Cavovarus feet with fixed hindfoot varus result in ulceration under the cuboid.

alignment is assessed on the axial intraoperatively views and corrected with additional lateral closing wedge ± translational calcaneal osteotomy (**Fig. 6**A and B).

Patients with negative coleman block test (stage 1B)
Progression of neuropathy results in variable degree of stiff hindfoot varus and plantar-flexed first ray. The treatment depending on the flexibility of the first ray and correction of tibio-calcaneal alignment as described above.

After the above correction, if the midfoot supination is noted, it is managed based on its flexibility with tibialis posterior tendon transfer or corrective bony osteotomies as described with stage 2.

Stage 2: neurologic cavovarus foot without hindfoot charcot neuroarthropathy
This stage is characterized by foot deformities similar to seen in patients with CMT, from weakness of the peroneal brevis and tibialis anterior muscle groups but exacerbated in patients with diabetic peripheral neuropathy with stiff hindfoot varus, midfoot apparent supination, adduction, and plantar-flexed first ray. The deformity progresses from being flexible to start with (Stage 2A) becoming rigid very quickly (Stage 2B). The bony architecture in this stage is maintained with no evidence of ankle CN.

The earliest clinical feature of this stage is the callus at the base of fifth metatarsal/cuboid (see **Fig. 1**). As the midfoot deformity progresses, this can break down to ulceration (see **Fig. 4**) or develop stress fracture of fifth metatarsal (see **Fig. 5**).

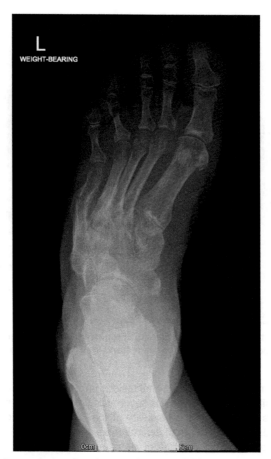

Fig. 5. Cavovarus foot associated with stress fracture of fifth metatarsal.

Additional callus or ulcerations can be seen under the big toe metatarsal head from the tightness of peroneal longus muscle group and under the middle metatarsal heads from additional tightness of gastroc-soleus-tendo-Achilles complex (see **Fig. 3**). Callosity with ulceration can be seen on the lateral border of the heel in patients with a plantigrade foot or following previous tendo-Achilles lengthening (TAL) (see **Fig. 1**). The intrinsic weakness induced claw toe deformity progresses as the motor neuropathy deteriorates resulting in tear of the plantar plate and worsening of forefoot plantar pressures.[6] This can lead to additional calluses followed by ulceration at the tips of the toes and dorsal surfaces of the proximal interphalangeal joints (PIPJ).

Progressive deformity with unprotected walking can result in early breakdown to ulceration and stress fractures. In addition, lateral ligament instability from attenuation of lateral ligaments result in progressive collapse of the medial body of talus and initiation of ankle CN (see **Fig. 8**).[20,21]

Treatment Options

Nonoperative treatment with custom orthosis or TCC can be considered in the pre-ulcerative stage, but rapid progression to ulceration without intervention is likely hence close monitoring is advised.[10] Before a planned surgical intervention, a period of

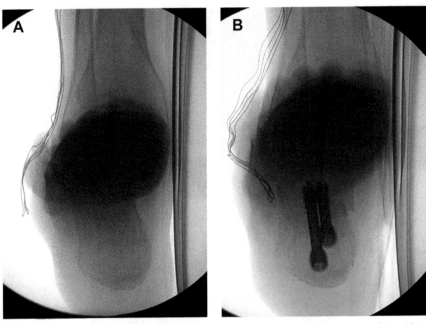

Fig. 6. (A and B) Intraoperative, preoperative, and postoperative radiographs of fixed hindfoot varus corrected with lateral closing wedge and translational osteotomy.

immobilization in the TCC might be beneficial for improving the skin and soft tissues around the callosities and improves the severity of ulceration. The surgical treatment of the deformities depends on the flexibility of the joints as guided by the Coleman block test, the presence and depth of ulceration as assessed by MR imaging, and preoperative CT assessment of bony deformities.

Patients with Flexible Joints and Positive Coleman Block Test (Stage 2A)

As with Stage 1, the procedure starts with peroneal tendon tenodesis ± percutaneous release of plantar fascia. Depending on the flexibility and correction of first ray, the Jones' transfer or proximal dorsal closing wedge osteotomy is advised. The hindfoot alignment is corrected with a lateral closing wedge ± translational calcaneal osteotomy (see **Fig. 6**A and B).

Once these deformities are corrected, apparent "flexible" midfoot supination deformity if persists, corrected with transfer of tibialis posterior tendon either in full or a split transfer to supplement the weak tibialis anterior muscle and the second part inserted into the cuboid.[7]

Patients with Rigid Deformities and Negative Coleman Block Test (Stage 2B)

The procedure starts with correction of hindfoot alignment, with a lateral closing wedge ± translational calcaneal osteotomy and in patients with severe deformity when the correction is thought to be inadequate additional soft tissue releases such as the deltoid ligament and z-lengthening of tibialis posterior tendon with its sheath helps to correct this axial deformity. If the ankle joint is noted to be unstable from the above releases and from attenuated lateral structures, a tibio-talar-calcaneal (TTC) joint fusion is recommended similar to Stage 3 disease as described below.

Once the hindfoot is corrected, the "fixed" midfoot apparent adduction and supination is corrected with a lateral column closing wedge + de-rotational osteotomy extending from the mid-cuboid up to the medial cuneiform, maintaining the integrity of the medial column. This closing wedge osteotomy is stabilized with a combination of a compression screw and a neutralization plate (**Fig. 7**A and B).

Ulceration or callus under the first metatarsal head is managed depending on the presence of local sepsis and intramedullary osteomyelitis as assessed on the preoperative MR imaging. As with the Stage 1, after a combination of peroneal tenodesis, release of distal peroneal longus tendon, and percutaneous plantar fascial release, a dorsal closing wedge metatarsal osteotomy is planned based on the residual plantar flexion and stabilized with a staple if there is no evidence of osteomyelitis. In the presence of osteomyelitis, the intramedullary canal is curetted and filled with local antibiotic eluting agent and the osteotomy stabilized with a percutaneous smooth wire extending from the tip of the toe to the first TMTJ.

The calluses or ulcerations under the middle metatarsal heads are managed with additional percutaneous or open distal TAL first, and if the metatarsal heads remain prominent, managed similarly with proximal metatarsal osteotomies based on the preoperative MR imaging findings of osteomyelitis. In patients who did not need a lateral closing wedge osteotomy, the distal plantar forefoot pressures are reduced with proximal metatarsal osteotomies or distal metaphyseal metatarsal osteotomies.

Patients with significant claw toe deformities with callosities or ulceration at the tip of the toes are managed depending on the flexibility of the toes. If some flexibility is noted, percutaneous flexor tenotomies reduce the pressures at the tips of the toes.

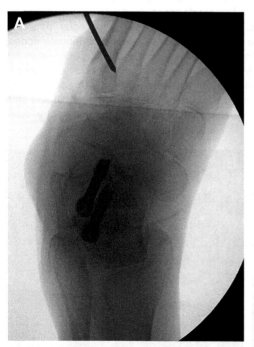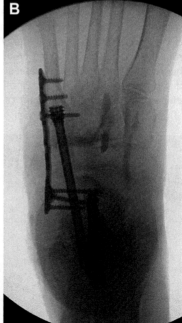

Fig. 7. (*A* and *B*) Intraoperative, preoperative, and postoperative radiographs of corrected midfoot adduction and protonation with lateral de-rotational closing wedge osteotomy stabilized with a lateral column compression screw and a neutralization plate.

This, however, does not correct the fixed flexion deformities at the PIPJ, which are corrected with PIPJ fusion stabilized with percutaneous 1.6 mm k-wire, removed at week 6.

Stage 3: rigid cavovarus feet with hindfoot charcot neuroarthropathy

As the fixed hindfoot varus progresses to ankle CN (see **Fig. 8**), additional callus with rapid progression to ulceration is noted under the prominent lateral malleolus, fractures of the shaft of fifth and less commonly of fourth metatarsals (see **Fig. 5**), and ulceration on the lateral border of the foot at the base of fifth metatarsal or cuboid.

Treatment Options

Nonoperative treatment with TCC has a high risk of ulceration at the prominent malleolus. As with Stage 2, a period of TCC preoperatively helps the soft tissues to settle and can help reduce the severity of ulcer.

Operative Treatment

A two-stage procedure is recommended in patients with an ulcer or osteomyelitis as noted on the preoperative MR imaging scan.

First Stage Specific to Stage 3 with Ulceration

If the patient has been on long-term antibiotics and are systemically well with normal inflammatory markers, all antibiotics are preferably stopped for a minimum of 14 days before the first stage procedure. Patient is positioned supine on the operating table, and the use of a thigh tourniquet is optional but is standard in authors practice except in patients who had venous bypass grafts. After standard prep of the surgical site, both the dorsalis pedis and posterior tibial vessels are marked with handheld Doppler and skin incisions are planned accordingly. A trans-lateral malleolar approach excising the involved segment of the lateral malleolus will provide adequate access to the ankle and subtalar joints. An additional anteromedial approach extending from the medial malleolus to first TMTJ (part or full) can give adequate access to the medial column. The ankle and subtalar alignment are corrected with a combination of soft tissue releases as described and corrective osteotomies of the tibia and talus after excising the diseased part of the talus with an aim to achieve a neutral tibio-

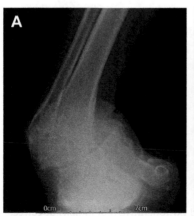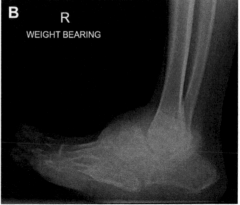

Fig. 8. (*A* and *B*) Stage 3 disease characterized by ankle Charcot neuroarthropathy with collapse of the body of talus and varus tibio-talar joint.

calcaneal alignment. The joints are adequately prepared, additional multiple drill holes help to curette the area of osteomyelitis and aid in joint preparation. Once adequate samples taken, the drill holes, the dead space, and the prepared joint surfaces are filled with local antibiotic eluting agents and the construct stabilized with either multiple thick threaded wires or external fixation. The postoperative course after the first stage is described in the earlier section.

During the second stage, the TTC joints are stabilized and fused with a TTC nail. The rigidity of the fixation construct is enhancing by achieving an isthmus fit of the hindfoot nail, additional de-rotational parallel calcaneo-tibial compression screw(s), and intact medial malleolus.[17,18] Additional midfoot CN deformity, if noted, is corrected with medially based wedge resections and stabilization with intramedullary beams and plates.[17,20,22] The postoperative course after the second stage is as described above.

SUMMARY

Neurologic cavovarus foot associated with diabetic peripheral neuropathy results in exacerbated and rapidly progressive foot and ankle deformity. This is flexible to start with but becomes rigid very quickly; hence, nonoperative treatment with a TCC or custom orthosis carries a high risk of ulceration under the bone prominences. The surgical treatment is based on the flexibility of the joints, as assessed by the Coleman block test and the degree of hindfoot stiffness and characteristics and progression of calluses. We describe three stages of the disease and provided the treatment strategy for each stage.

Cavovarus foot deformity in patients with complicated diabetes is best managed by an MDFT. Preoperative medical and vascular optimization and adjustment to home micro-environment are critical for a successful outcome following surgical correction. Deformity correction followed by stabilization with an internal or external fixation method can be chosen based on surgeon's preference and the stages of the disease. The internal fixation method is the preferred option for the authors as it provides an excellent opportunity to correct the deformity with higher fusion rates and low and acceptable complication rates.[11,13,20]

CLINICS CARE POINTS

- A subtle cavovarus foot deformity is a common non-familial and non-neurological foot deformity, characterised by 'peek-a-boo' sign.
- Patients with subtle cavovarus foot deformity commonly presents with history of recurrent ankle sprains and in patients with diabetic peripheral neuropathy, callus under the first metatarsal head.
- Coleman block test assess the flexibility of subtalar joint and guide the treatment in patients with non-neurological cavovarus foot deformity.
- Callus/ ulceration under the middle metatarsal heads is due to the tightness of gastrocsoleus-tendo-Achilles complex, while the tightness of peroneus longus results in callus /ulceration under the first metatarsal head while the tightness of tibialis posterior results in callus /ulceration under the 5th metatarsal head.

DISCLOSURE

The authors have nothing to disclose.

REFERENCES

1. Seaman TJ, Ball TA, Pes Cavus. [Updated 2022 Aug 8]. In: StatPearls [Internet]. Treasure Island (FL): StatPearls Publishing; 2023. Available at: https://www.ncbi.nlm.nih.gov/books/NBK556016/.

2. Ward CM, Dolan LA, Bennett DL, et al. Long-term results of reconstruction for treatment of a flexible cavovarus foot in Charcot-Marie-Tooth disease. J Bone Joint Surg Am 2008;90(12):2631–42.

3. Leeuwesteijn AE, de Visser E, Louwerens JW. Flexible cavovarus feet in Charcot-Marie-Tooth disease treated with first ray proximal dorsiflexion osteotomy combined with soft tissue surgery: a short-term to mid-term outcome study. Foot Ankle Surg 2010;16(3):142–7.

4. Kołodziej L, Dobiecki K, Sadlik B. Surgical treatment of advanced, stiff neurologic cavovarus foot in adults. Ortop Traumatol Rehabil 2013;15(4):325–33.

5. Mansour AA, Dahyak SG. Are foot abnormalities more common in adults with diabetes? A cross-sectional study in basrah, Iraq. Perm J 2008;12(4):25–30.

6. Kimura T, Thorhauer ED, Kindig MW, et al. Neuropathy, claw toes, intrinsic muscle volume, and plantar aponeurosis thickness in diabetic feet. BMC Musculoskelet Disord 2020;21(1):485.

7. Deben SE, Pomeroy GC. Subtle cavus foot: diagnosis and management. J Am Acad Orthop Surg 2014;22(8):512–20.

8. Coleman SS, Chesnut WJ. A simple test for hindfoot flexibility in the cavovarus foot. Clin Orthop Relat Res 1977;123:60–2.

9. Grant WP, Sullivan R, Sonenshine DE, et al. Electron microscopic investigation of the effects of diabetes mellitus on the Achilles tendon. J Foot Ankle Surg 1997; 36(4):272–8.

10. Armstrong DG, Boulton AJM, Bus SA. Diabetic Foot Ulcers and Their Recurrence. N Engl J Med 2017;376(24):2367–75.

11. Kavarthapu V, Vris A. Charcot midfoot reconstruction- surgical technique based on deformity patterns. Ann Joint 2020;5:28.

12. Laborde JM. Neuropathic plantar forefoot ulcers treated with tendon lengthenings. Foot Ankle Int 2008;29(4):378–84.

13. Kavarthapu V, Budair B. Two-stage reconstruction of infected Charcot foot using internal fixation. Bone Joint Lett J 2021;103-B(10):1611–8.

14. Wukich DK, Joseph A, Ryan M, et al. Outcomes of ankle fractures in patients with uncomplicated versus complicated diabetes. Foot Ankle Int 2011;32(2):120–30.

15. Lavery LA, Armstrong DG, Harkless LB. Classification of diabetic foot wounds. J Foot Ankle Surg 1996;35(6):528–31.

16. Ahluwalia R, Vainieri E, Tam J, et al. Surgical Diabetic Foot Debridement: Improving Training and Practice Utilizing the Traffic Light Principle. Int J Low Extrem Wounds 2019;18(3):279–86.

17. Sammarco VJ. Superconstructs in the treatment of charcot foot deformity: plantar plating, locked plating, and axial screw fixation. Foot Ankle Clin 2009;14(3): 393–407.

18. Pisters R, Lane DA, Nieuwlaat R, et al. A novel user-friendly score (HAS-BLED) to assess 1-year risk of major bleeding in patients with atrial fibrillation: the Euro Heart Survey. Chest 2010;138(5):1093–100.

19. Paulos L, Coleman SS, Samuelson KM. Pes cavovarus. Review of a surgical approach using selective soft-tissue procedures. J Bone Joint Surg Am 1980; 62(6):942–53.

20. Kavarthapu V, Guduri V, Hester T. Combined Charcot hindfoot and midfoot reconstruction using internal fixation method—surgical technique and single surgeon series. Ann Joint 2023;8:10.
21. Kavarthapu V, Hester T. Charcot hindfoot deformity reconstruction using a hindfoot nail- surgical technique. J Clin Orthop Trauma 2021;16:277–84.
22. Butt DA, Hester T, Bilal A, et al. The medial column Synthes Midfoot Fusion Bolt is associated with unacceptable rates of failure in corrective fusion for Charcot deformity: Results from a consecutive case series. Bone Joint Lett J 2015; 97-B(6):809–13.

Nonneurologic Cavovarus Feet in Skeletally Immature Patients
Main Causes and Principles of Treatment

Jordanna Maria Pereira Bergamasco, MD*,
Noé De Marchi Neto, MD, Marco Túlio Costa, MD

KEYWORDS

- Metatarsal • Cavovarus • Charcot-marie-tooth • Subtalar sprains

KEY POINTS

- Cavus foot, defined as a highly arched foot, is not infrequent in childhood and is an asymptomatic normal foot variant.
- Cavovarus foot denotes the presence of a three-dimensional deformity of the foot, but it is much more a descriptive feature than a diagnosis.
- Isolated injuries to nerves, muscles, and tendons can result in cavovarus foot and may provide insight into how specific muscle imbalance can cause a foot deformity.
- Less common nonneurological causes of cavus are skeletal dysplasia syndromes, birth defects, progression of congenital idiopathic clubfoot, tarsal coalition, and trauma.

INTRODUCTION

The foot resembles a tripod. The 3 legs consist of (1) the tip of the heel, (2) the first metatarsal (1MMT), and (3) the fifth metatarsal. This concept is useful to explain cavus or flat feet. When the tips of the tripod move closer, the arch becomes higher. The leg of the tripod that moves the most will determine the type of cavus feet, which can be hindfoot cavus, forefoot cavus, or 1MMT cavus.

Cavus foot is defined as a highly arched foot, is not infrequent in childhood, and is an asymptomatic normal foot variant. However, certain forms of cavus, such as pes cavovarus (PCV) or pes calcaneocavus, may be related to a neurologic lesion and its secondary muscle imbalance and may be symptomatic.[1] Because of the multiple causes and a varying severity of cavus foot, the natural history may not be predictable. Cavovarus is defined as plantar flexion of the forefoot with associated hindfoot varus.[2]

Foot and Ankle Group, Santa Casa de Misericórdia de São Paulo, 916 Angélica Avenue, (608) São Paulo - Brazil 01228-000
* Corresponding author.
E-mail address: drajordannabergamasco@gmail.com

Foot Ankle Clin N Am 28 (2023) 889–901
https://doi.org/10.1016/j.fcl.2023.05.007
foot.theclinics.com

Cavovarus foot denotes the presence of a three-dimensional deformity of the foot, but it is much more a descriptive feature than a diagnosis. Although PCV may be idiopathic in origin, in most cases, there is an underlying neurologic condition. Therefore, one of the most important challenges is to elucidate the responsible cause for the deformity. Finding the correct diagnosis can be difficult, often beyond the scope of an orthopedic surgeon, and usually a neuropediatric colleague may help conduct the case. However, the search for the cause should never be ignored: first, because the nature of the condition may determine the quality and life expectancy of the patient, and second, because the authors' management plan will largely depend on the subsequent diagnosis.[1]

The true incidence of cavovarus feet is unknown. There are reports suggesting that its presence increases with age, ranging from a 2% presence at 3 years of age to up to a 7% presence at the age of 16 years,[3] although the incidence could be much higher in the adult population, ranging from 10.5% to 25%.[4]

Population-based studies suggest the prevalence of cavus feet is approximately 10% to 20%, some of which represent a normal variant. Around 66% of cavovarus feet are the result of subtle neurologic diseases and conditions that may not become clinically evident until later in life. Generally, the cause can be attributed to the brain, spinal cord, peripheral nerves, or muscular/structural problems of the foot. Two-thirds of adults with a symptomatic cavus foot have an underlying neurologic condition, the most common being Charcot-Marie-Tooth (CMT) disease. In cases of unknown causes, it can be considered "idiopathic"; however, those labeled idiopathic may likely be the result of a very subtle neurologic lesion below clinical detection.[2]

Although the number of neurologic conditions that may lead to cavus foot is extensive, the common factor is muscle imbalance that disrupts the synergy between the intrinsic and extrinsic muscles. Nonneurologic causes are less common; they include skeletal dysplasia syndromes, birth defects, progression of congenital idiopathic clubfoot, tarsal coalition, and trauma. Idiopathic PCV is exceedingly rare[5] (**Box 1**).

Isolated injuries to nerves, muscles, and tendons can result in cavovarus foot and may provide insight into how specific muscle imbalance can cause a foot deformity. Cavus deformity may occur after an injection injury to the sciatic nerve,[6] after fibrous contracture of the deep posterior compartment resulting from vascular damage, can be a missed deep compartment syndrome, or a severe muscle laceration, or a combination of these mechanisms. Cavovarus deformity has also been associated with clubfoot or residual clubfoot deformity in 22% of children.[6,7]

An understanding of the underlying muscle imbalance in the cavovarus foot is extremely important to guide treatment.[5] Flexible cavovarus feet in children and adolescents can be very challenging, especially those that get worse with growth. A

Box 1
Non-neurologic causes of cavovarus feet

1. Muscular dystrophies
2. Posttraumatic
3. Secondary to vascular ischemia and compartmental syndrome
4. Secondary to clubfoot
5. Associated to syndromes
6. Idiopathic

careful history and physical examination are Primordial for determining the best treatment strategy, but a multitude of options are available. Specific treatment strategies must be individualized, and any bony correction has to be in association with a muscle-balancing procedure.[2]

Treating the deformity in the immature skeleton has the advantage of bone remodeling when muscle balance is achieved, but with the potential for growth, undercorrections may lead to recurrence of the deformities. Excessive pressure on the head of the 1MMT or base of the fifth metatarsal during weight-bearing may cause pain; usually children tolerate it well, but it can become disabling in adults. For these reasons, nonneurologic cases should be treated early. Ankle instability may manifest as recurrent tibiotarsal or subtalar sprains (hindfoot varus and weakness of the peroneus brevis muscle). Persistence of these abnormalities may result in chronic ankle instability, which has a severe impact on functional outcomes and progression of the deformity[8] and cause pain and disability in adulthood.

PHYSICAL EXAMINATION

Clinical examination should include a shoeless assessment of the patient's gait. In younger children, the physical examination often ends up being complicated, and the help of parents is essential. As most cases have neurologic causes, the clinical examination needs to include a thorough neurologic evaluation and a complete clinical history in search of congenital malformations that could cause such deformities.

The presence of a foot drop or an extensor recruitment to compensate for weak dorsiflexion should be noted, and again, in the youngest, it might be quite challenging. Abnormal heel and tandem walking may be an early sign of alert. When a calcaneocavus foot is present, a peg-leg gait may appear as a result of the poor push-off. The Trendelenburg test should be included in the dynamic assessment.[1]

It is important to check side involvement unilaterally or bilaterally (**Fig. 1**); assess the hindfoot position and differentiate between the type of cavus deformity, as well as assess the flexibility of the hindfoot, using the Coleman block test.[9] In the Coleman test, the patient is asked to stand with the heel and lateral border of the foot over a 2 centimeters block while the medial metatarsals contact the floor. When the hindfoot is flexible, the heel will return to a neutral or valgus position.[10]

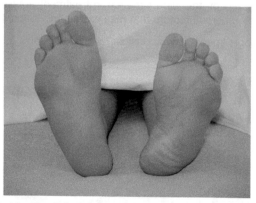

Fig. 1. A 7-year-old girl with a left cavovarus foot. No neurologic problem was found in the diagnostic investigation.

The clinical evaluation must identify the apex of the deformity, and search for other foot anomalies: assessing associated toes deformities is an example; assessing where callosities are present, usually at the head of the first and fifth and base of the fifth metatarsals, and lateral side of the hindfoot; assessing the flexibility of the foot joints and whether a manual correction of the deformities is possible; assessing ankle mobility, especially in the older ones and adolescents, and also assess the Achilles length.[1]

A global examination should include the following: a detailed spine examination looking for hairy patches, dimples, or structural deformities; and hip assessment, including motion (to exclude hip dysplasia). Finally, the hands should be evaluated for wasting of the intrinsic muscles (thinking on CMT). A basic neurologic examination should include muscle power, with good attention to the evertors, tendon reflexes, and a sensory examination.[1]

RADIOGRAPHIC EVALUATION

The standard measurements for foot deformity should include the following:

1. Meary angle (normal value: 0°): The longitudinal axis of the 1MTT and the talus normally forms a straight line. When a cavus foot is present, the lines intersect at the apex of the deformity (normally at the dorsal aspect of the first cuneiform body). An increase is indicative of 1MTT plantar flexion (**Fig. 2**).
2. Calcaneal pitch is the angle formed by a line along the plantar surface of the os calcis and a line that goes through the floor. The normal value is less than 25°. A calcaneal pitch greater than 30° is indicative of posterior cavus (calcaneocavus).
3. Hibbs angle is formed by a line through the calcaneus and the axis of the 1MTT. Normal value is less than 45°.
4. AP-talus-1MTT angle (12 abduction, −10 adduction). In a normal foot, the line formed by the longitudinal axis of the talus and the 1MTT is parallel or intersects at the body or neck of the talus.[11] In malalignment, the axes intersect at the level of talonavicular or the head of the talus. The 1MTT is always adducted in relation to the talus.

MANAGING NONNEUROLOGIC CAVOVARUS FEET

There is a lack of consensus about what constitutes the ideal treatment for cavovarus feet, which is reflected by the wide variation in treatment applied in different centers.[12,13] There are numerous factors that may explain this disparity.

1. The wide aetiologic spectrum responsible for this deformity,

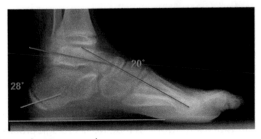

Fig. 2. Lateral radiograph, Meary angle.

2. The variable severity of involvement even in patients sharing a common mutation, and finally, and even more importantly,
3. The paucity of long-term reports describing the various techniques.[8]

Another factor rarely discussed in the literature is that of the differences in treatment between children and adults. Many studies report adults and children together, making no stratification of the results according to age. The importance of segregating these populations lies in the fact that muscle imbalance in children occurs in a growing skeleton; therefore, the uneven forces will favor a skewed bone growth and an abnormal development of the bony structures. Nonneurologic cases should be treated as soon as possible, seeking muscle balance so that the cartilaginous model ossifies in a better position.[1,5]

Conservative treatment has been recommended in the nonprogressive flexible cavovarus foot, as insoles supporting the lateral side of the foot or with metatarsal bars, unloading the areas of excessive pressure. Other therapies, such as stretching, activity modification, and modified footwear, have also been described.[2,14,15] Trials with the use of Botulin toxin have proven ineffective.[11] A French group proposed the use of casting and night splinting until achieving skeletal maturity, which showed a modest beneficial result,[16] but it requires much adherence to the treatment and collaboration of the parents. The children the authors treat in their practice have few resources, come from large families with many children, and the parents end up not being able to follow treatments that require a great deal of dedication.

The objectives of a successful treatment are to achieve a painless, plantigrade, mobile foot.

The principles of treatment of PCV laid down by Mosca in 2001[16] are still applicable.

1. Correct all of the segmental deformities while preserving motion,
2. Balance the remaining forces,
3. Leave reasonable treatment options available for possible recurrence of deformity and pain.[17]

As the causes of cavovarus feet are numerous and treatments must be selected according to the causes, the authors have separated the most common causes of nonneurologic cavovarus feet in skeletally immature patients, and a little about each of them is detailed in later discussion.

Congenital Clubfoot

Idiopathic congenital clubfoot (ICCF) is a foot deformity characterized by hindfoot varus, forefoot adductus, an augmented midfoot arch, and equinus, and its cause is largely unknown.

Congenital clubfoot or talipes equinovarus is one of the most common pediatric deformities: 0.5 to 2.0 cases per 1000 live births, which results in an estimated 7 to 43 cases of clubfoot per year per million population, depending mainly on the birth rate.[18]

The ICCF is a complex three-dimensional congenital malformation that affects the lower limb, causing deformities that are identified at birth or have later appearance. The deformities result from the muscle imbalance between strong inverting and weak evertor muscles.[19] Several treatments have been proposed throughout the centuries, but today, the gold-standard treatment is the Ponseti method.[20]

Ponseti first described his treatment regime including abduction bracing and tibialis anterior tendon transfer for the treatment of relapse in 1963 and published a further detailed description in 1972.[19,20] All recommendations are still valid today, and only minor adjustments have been made over the decades. The superior results of his method were reported by Ponseti himself and his colleagues in a different long-term study.[20]

The method consists of short and gentle manipulation before casting. This manipulation is important to stretch the structures and additionally to get a feeling for the flexibility of the foot and the amount of correction that can be achieved with the cast. Serial casting is performed with above-the-knee casts because short leg casts cannot hold the abduction and frequently slip off. In the first cast, the 1MMT must be raised, which means supinating the forefoot to align it with the hindfoot and to decrease cavus. The foot should never be pronated. In the following casts, a pure abduction with counterpressure on the neck of the talus is performed (**Fig. 3**). Thereby, the talus is stabilized and cannot rotate in the ankle mortise, while the rest of the foot is abducted underneath it. The calcaneus must not be touched, as this might block the motion of the calcaneus, which must be free to swing out from underneath the talus and thereby abducts, everts, and dorsiflexes. Active dorsiflexion must not be performed before the subtalar joint is fully corrected.[21] In the authors' practice, they routinely manipulate the feet for 5 to 10 minutes before casting.

Ponseti recommended a thin cast with only a little padding, which should be very well molded onto the foot. The authors usually use flannel fabric as padding to prevent irritation on children's skin. In addition, the crease above the heel must be well molded, and the cast must reach high enough to the groin with the knee in at least 90° of flexion and with the cast molded well around and behind the knee, to prevent slipping of the cast. Slipping of the cast has been recognized to be a major factor in the development of recurrence and complex club foot.[21]

A tenotomy should be performed early with about 30° to 40° of abduction, and foot abduction bracing should be started in the same abduction as achieved in the last cast (**Fig. 4**).

In all cases, cast removal should only be performed just before a new cast is applied, as it has been shown that removing the cast the night before results in a higher number of casts being necessary for correction.[22] The authors usually remove it with a gentle saw minutes before starting the manipulation. Parents use these few minutes to clean up the children.

Cast changes are typically done once a week, but accelerated protocols have been reported.[22] Morcuende and colleague described similar results with cast changes every 5 days.[22,23] Another study group reported cast changes 3 times per week and

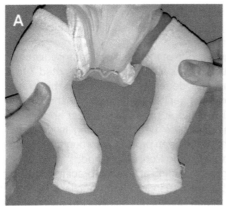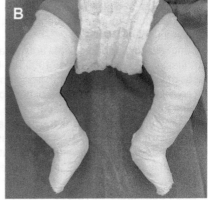

Fig. 3. (A) First cast to correct the cavus deformity. (B) Third cast for abduction.

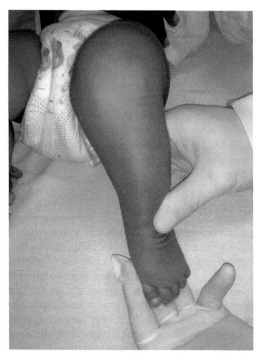

Fig. 4. Congenital clubfoot treated by the Ponseti method, with the abduction obtained before the Achilles tendon lengthening.

again found similar results compared with a standard weekly cast change group.[24] In the authors' practice, they carry out the manipulation and cast changes every 7 days.

The authors advocate starting treatment as early as possible. In their practice, the authors start as soon as the child leaves maternity. Others suggested that casting should be postponed until after the first 4 weeks of life or until the foot reaches a length of at least 8 cm to make casting easier. Nevertheless, there seems to be a consensus that treatment for club foot should start not later than within the first month of life.[25]

To monitor the treatment progress and to help in finding the right time for the percutaneous Achilles tenotomy as well as for scoring the foot at presentation, the Pirani score has been introduced with very good interobserver reliability and ease of use.[26] Although a study found only a low correlation of the score at presentation with the number of Ponseti casts required for correction, significant correlation was reported between initial severity of the foot and outcomes.[26] The authors have about 300 registered cases, and in their perception, the Pirani classification did not show a direct relationship with the number of casts or with a worse prognosis.

Over the past 2 decades, the Ponseti "conservative" (nonsurgical) method of clubfoot treatment has been adopted worldwide. As a result, the need for operative treatment for clubfoot has decreased dramatically. However, even Ponseti himself routinely used surgery for certain patients: at least 90% of feet need percutaneous tenotomy, and 15% to 40% may require tibialis anterior tendon transfer.[27]

Treatment should start early to obtain a plantigrade foot for the development of gait. However, even in the initially corrected feet, the excessive synthesis of collagen in the posterior and medial ligaments and tendons causes adduction and supination deformities to appear later, as the child grows and develops gait, and may progress until 3 or 4 years of age.[28] Regardless of the method applied to correct the initial ICCF deformities, recurrence happens in 0.6% to 53.3% of the cases.[19,28]

There is still no consensus on the cause or causes of recurrence: whether it is due to a natural history of the deformity, the nonadherence of orthotic treatment after manipulations or after the initial correction, and the identification and/or the appearance of muscle imbalance between the anterior tibialis tendon (stronger) and the peroneal tendons (weaker).[29] Recent studies have increasingly emphasized the degree of muscle imbalance present and show a positive correlation between relapse rates and weakness of the evertor muscles.[28,30]

RESIDUAL CLUBFOOT DEFORMITIES

In the authors' outpatient practice, they often find nonneurologic cavovarus feet in patients with neglected recurrent congenital clubfeet (**Fig. 5**). The first choice for residual clubfoot deformity, even in the case of older children, is another series of casting before considering surgery. For a persistent cavovarus deformity in children older than 3 years of age, indications for tendon transfer and/or osteotomies are good options.[31] It is not easy to define the right moment to indicate bone correction with osteotomies. On one hand, there is much potential for growth, and an adequate muscle balance can provide a more aligned bone development; however, some structured deformities do not present complete correction with muscle balance, even in younger children with great growth potential (**Fig. 6**).

It is very important to differentiate a dynamic supination from a cavovarus deformity. In a dynamic supination case, the tibialis anterior transfer is a successful operation.

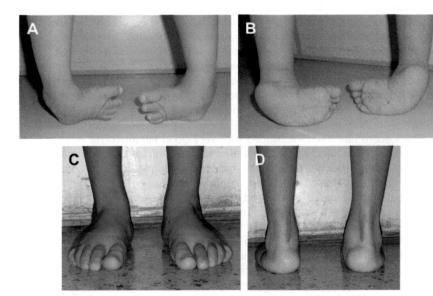

Fig. 5. A 4-year-old boy with neglected bilateral congenital clubfoot. (*A*) Anterior view. (*B*) Posterior view. (*C*) Two years after Ponseti method, Achilles tendon lengthening, and anterior tibial tendon transfer, anterior view. (*D*) Posterior view.

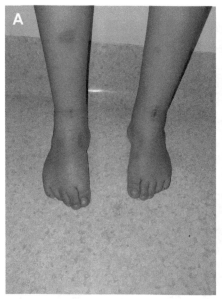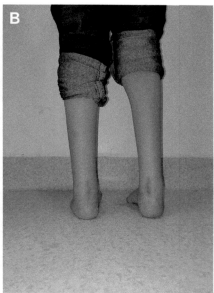

Fig. 6. A 7-year-old boy, bilateral congenital clubfoot treated by the Ponseti method, missed follow-up, showed recurrence of the deformities, after 4 years, resumed Ponseti, and underwent an anterior tibial tendon transfer, but 3 years after surgery showed up with a cavo varus deformity again. (*A*) Anterior view. (*B*) Posterior view.

The transfer can be performed as soon the ossified nucleus of the lateral cuneiform is visible at the age of 3 to 4 years, or later, after the maturation of the inverter muscles.[32] However, a residual cavovarus deformity might be treated by plantar fascia release and selective tendon transfer or 1MMT osteotomy according to patients with CMT, with the advantage that these deformities are not progressive, which ensures a more predictable and lasting result.

TARSAL COALITION

Another (not so common) cause of cavovarus feet is the tarsal coalition. Tarsal coalition is defined as absence of segmentation between 2 or more foot bones during embryologic development owing to failure of the joint cleft to develop. Depending on the nature of the connecting tissue (which may change during growth), the coalition is a syndesmosis, synchondrosis, or synostosis.

Although tarsal coalition is present at birth, ossification of the connecting tissue (synostosis) usually occurs later on.[33] Tarsal coalition is both a malformation, because one or more tarsal joints are lacking, and a deformity, because hindfoot valgus or varus often develops secondarily.[33]

Talocalcaneal coalition may affect the arch of the foot. Coalition involving the middle facet is usually associated with pes planus, whereas cavus feet may be present in patients with posterior facet coalition.[34]

The diagnosis is often made at symptom onset, which often coincides with ossification of the coalition during the second decade of life. Pain during physical activities and efforts is the main symptom. Motion range abolition or restriction should be sought during the physical examination. Rigid flatfoot with valgus deformity is typical, but varus deformity or cavus feet may be also seen.[34]

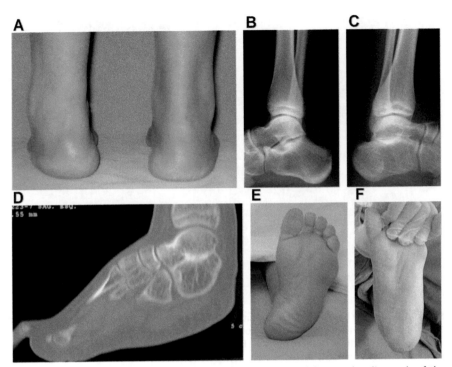

Fig. 7. (*A*) A 12-year-old girl with a left cavovarus deformity. (*B*) Lateral radiograph of the right foot. (*C*) Lateral radiograph of the left foot with a subtalar coalition. (*D*) Subtalar coalition. (*E*) Preoperative deformity. (*F*) Postoperative correction, calcaneal osteotomy.

Patients usually begin to present symptoms in early adolescence, and diagnostic investigation should begin with a radiographic study. A standard oblique radiograph ensures the diagnosis of calcaneonavicular synostosis, whereas computed tomography (CT) and MRI are the investigations of choice for diagnosing talocalcaneal synostosis. The presence of secondary signs suggesting synostosis should lead to investigation by CT or MRI.

Pes planus or cavus feet is not a contraindication to resection, but the associated deformity should also be corrected if possible.[34] Tarsal coalition does not cause pain until the second decade of life or adulthood. As the coalition ossifies over time, leading to synostosis, the range of motion diminishes, and the pain worsens. Synostosis is thought to induce degenerative changes with advancing age.[35] The more ossified the foot is at the time of resection, the greater the need for correction of associated deformities. Thus, the authors believe that as soon as the symptoms appear, if conservative treatment with analgesia and rest does not resolve, surgery should be indicated. In cases of more severe deformities, the authors always associate corrective osteotomies to the resection of the synostosis (**Fig. 7**).

POSTTRAUMATIC CAVOVARUS FEET

Some traumas and fractures in the foot and ankle result in a cavovarus deformity. Among the fractures, the fracture of the neck of the talus can consolidate in varus and evolve with the deformity. Other causes of residual cavovarus deformity include burns, sequelae of compartment syndrome, and injury to the peroneal tendons (**Fig. 8**).

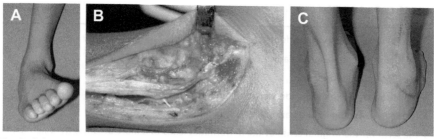

Fig. 8. (*A*) A 9-year-old boy with a history of an accident in a glass window presenting with a cut in the lateral side of the right ankle 1 year ago, evolved with a hindfoot varus deformity. (*B*) Intraoperative image of injured peroneal tendon repair with extensor digitorum longus graft. (*C*) 6 months after surgery.

Fractures of the talus have been described to be rare injuries with an incidence of 0.08% in the pediatric population (**Fig. 9**) compared with 0.3% in adults. Osteonecrosis and posttraumatic malalignment with subsequent arthritis represent the most significant complication[35]; however, Blount's claim from 1977 that the child's foot is very flexible and resilient[36] explains why such fractures are rarer in children and present less complications. The more immature the skeleton, the greater the ability to remodel.

FINAL CONSIDERATIONS

The main causes of cavovarus feet are attributed to neurologic conditions. Nonneurologic causes in skeletally immature patients include congenital clubfeet, tarsal coalition, and posttraumatic conditions.

Unlike neurologic cases, treatment must be applied early and usually presents good results with muscle balance and corrective osteotomies. Knowing the original cause of the deformity leads to a more accurate treatment with better results.

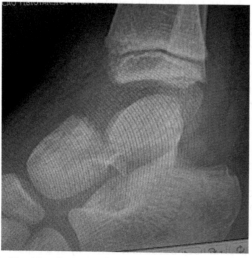

Fig. 9. A 5-year-old girl with a fracture of the talar neck.

CLINICS CARE POINTS

In non neurological cavovarus foot:

- treatment must be applied early.
- usually the results are good.
- muscle imbalance must be adressed with tendon transfers.
- corrective osteotomies are part of the therapeutic arsenal.
- the serch for the original cause of the defformities leads to a more accurate treatment and better results.

DISCLOSURE

None of the authors have any conflict of interest.

REFERENCES

1. Sanpera I, Villafranca-Solano S, Muñoz-Lopez C, et al. How to manage pes cavus in children and adolescents? EFORT Open Rev 2021;6(6):510–7.
2. VanderHave KL, Hensinger RN, King BW. Flexible cavovarus foot in children and adolescents. Foot Ankle Clin 2013;18(4):715–26.
3. Reimers J, Pedersen B, Brodersen A. Foot deformity and the length of the triceps surae in Danish children between 3 and 17 years old. J Pediatr Orthop B 1995; 4:71–3.
4. Aminian A, Sangeorzan BJ. The anatomy of cavus foot deformity. Foot Ankle Clin 2008;13:191–8, v.
5. Wicart p. Cavus foot, from neonates to adolescents. Orthop Traumatol Surg Res 2012;98:813–28.
6. Lee MC, Sucato DJ. Pediatric issues with cavovarus foot deformities. Foot Ankle Clin 2008;13:199–219.
7. Morcuende JA, Dolan LA, Dietz FR, et al. Radical reduction in the rate of extensive corrective surgery for clubfoot using the Ponseti method. Pediatrics 2004; 113(2):376–80.
8. Ward CM, Dolan LA, Bennett L, et al. Long-term results of reconstruction for treatment of a flexible cavovarus foot in Charcot-Marie-Tooth disease. J Bone Joint Surg 2008;90A:2631–42.
9. Mubarak sJ, Van Valin sE. Osteotomies of the foot for cavus deformities in children. J Pediatr Orthop 2009;29:294–9.
10. Wicart P, Seringe R. Plantar opening-wedge osteotomy of cuneiform bones combined with selective plantar release and Dwyer osteotomy for pes cavovarus in children. J Pediatr Orthop 2006;26:100–8.
11. D'astorg H, Rampal V, Seringe R, et al. Is non-operative management of childhood neurologic cavovarus foot effective? Orthop Traumatol Surg Res 2016; 102:1087–91.
12. Weiner DS, Jones K, Jonah D, et al. Management of the rigid cavus foot in children and adolescents. Foot Ankle Clin 2013;18:727–41.
13. Ziebarth K, Krause F. Updates in pediatric cavovarus deformity. Foot Ankle Clin 2019;24:205–17.
14. Schwend rM, Drennan JC. Cavus foot deformity in children. J Am Acad Orthop Surg 2003;11:201–11.

15. Burns J, Scheinberg A, Ryan MM, et al. Randomized trial of botulinum toxin to prevent pes cavus progression in pediatric Charcot–Marie–Tooth disease type 1A. Muscle Nerve 2010;42:262–7.
16. Mosca VS. The cavus foot. J Pediatr Orthop 2001;21:423–4.
17. Cooper DM, Dietz FR. Treatment of idiopathic club foot: a thirty-year follow-up note. J Bone Joint Surg 1995. Am 77-A:1477–1489.
18. Bergamasco JMP, Costa MT, Ferreira RC, et al. Anterior tibial tendon transfer in idiopathic clubfoot: does the outcome differ with the initial treatment? Proposed classification to surgical indication. Int Orthop 2022;46(6):1361–6.
19. Radler C. The Ponseti method for the treatment of congenital club foot: review of the current literature and treatment recommendations. Int Orthop 2013;37(9): 1747–53.
20. Ponseti IV, Zhivkov M, Davis N, et al. Treatment of the complex idiopathic club foot. Clin Orthop Relat Res 2006;451:171–6.
21. Terrazas-Lafargue G, Morcuende JA. Effect of cast removal timing in the correction of idiopathic club foot by the Ponseti method. Iowa Orthop J 2007;27:24–7.
22. Morcuende JA, Abbasi D, Dolan LA, et al. Results of an accelerated Ponseti protocol for club foot. J Pediatr Orthop 2005;25:623–6.
23. Harnett P, Freeman R, Harrison WJ, et al. An accelerated Ponseti versus the standard Ponseti method: a prospective randomised controlled trial. J Bone Joint Surg Br 2011;93(3):404–8.
24. Bohm S, Sinclair M. Report of the 1st European consensus meeting on Ponseti club foot treatment. J Child Orthop 2013;7(3):251–4.
25. Dyer PJ, Davis N. The role of the Pirani scoring system in the management of club foot by the Ponseti method. J Bone Joint Surg Br 2006;88(8):1082–4.
26. Eidelman M, Kotlarsky P, Herzenberg JE. Treatment of relapsed, residual and neglected clubfoot: adjunctive surgery. J Child Orthop 2019;13(3):293–303.
27. Gelfer Y, Dunkley M, Jackson D, et al. Evertor muscle activity as a predictor of the mid-term outcome following treatment of the idiopathic and non-idiopathic clubfoot. Bone Joint Lett J 2014;96-B(9):1264–8.
28. Kuo KN, Hennigan SP, Hastings ME. Anterior tibial transfer in residual dynamic clubfoot deformity. J Pediatr Orthop 2001;21(1):35–41.
29. Banskota B, Banskota AK, Regmi R, et al. The Ponseti method in the treatment of children with idiopathic clubfoot presenting between five and ten years of age. Bone Joint Lett J 2013;95-B(12):1721–5.
30. Dragoni M, Farsetti P, Vena G, et al. Ponseti treatment of rigid residual deformity in congenital clubfoot after walking age. J Bone Joint Surg Am 2016;98(20): 1706–12.
31. Ziebarth K, Krause F. Updates in Pediatric Cavovarus Deformity. Foot Ankle Clin 2019;24(2):205–17.
32. Mosca VS. Subtalar coalition in pediatrics. Foot Ankle Clin 2015;20:265–81.
33. Docquier PL, Maldaque P, Bouchard M. Tarsal coalition in paediatric patients. Orthop Traumatol Surg Res 2019;105(1S):S123–31.
34. Murphy JS, Mubarak SJ. Talocalcaneal coalitions. Foot Ankle Clin 2015;20: 681–91.
35. Eberl R, Singer G, Schalamon J, et al. Fractures of the talus - differences between children and adolescents. J Trauma 2010;68(1):126–30.
36. Blount WP. Fractures in children. Huntington, NY: Robert E. Krieger; 1977.

UNITED STATES POSTAL SERVICE®
Statement of Ownership, Management, and Circulation
(All Periodicals Publications Except Requester Publications)

1. Publication Title	2. Publication Number	3. Filing Date
FOOT AND ANKLE CLINICS OF NORTH AMERICA	016 – 368	9/18/2023

4. Issue Frequency	5. Number of Issues Published Annually	6. Annual Subscription Price
MAR, JUN, SEP, DEC	4	$362.00

7. Complete Mailing Address of Known Office of Publication (Not printer) (Street, city, county, state, and ZIP+4®)

ELSEVIER INC.
230 Park Avenue, Suite 800
New York, NY 10169

Contact Person
Malathi Samayan

Telephone (Include area code)
91-44-4299-4507

8. Complete Mailing Address of Headquarters or General Business Office of Publisher (Not printer)

ELSEVIER INC.
230 Park Avenue, Suite 800
New York, NY 10169

9. Full Names and Complete Mailing Addresses of Publisher, Editor, and Managing Editor (Do not leave blank)

Publisher (Name and complete mailing address)

DOLORES MELONI, ELSEVIER INC.
1600 JOHN F KENNEDY BLVD. SUITE 1600
PHILADELPHIA, PA 19103-2899

Editor (Name and complete mailing address)

MEGAN ASHDOWN, ELSEVIER INC.
1600 JOHN F KENNEDY BLVD. SUITE 1600
PHILADELPHIA, PA 19103-2899

Managing Editor (Name and complete mailing address)

PATRICK MANLEY, ELSEVIER INC.
1600 JOHN F KENNEDY BLVD. SUITE 1600
PHILADELPHIA, PA 19103-2899

10. Owner (Do not leave blank. If the publication is owned by a corporation, give the name and address of the corporation immediately followed by the names and addresses of all stockholders owning or holding 1 percent or more of the total amount of stock. If not owned by a corporation, give the names and addresses of the individual owners. If owned by a partnership or other unincorporated firm, give its name and address as well as those of each individual owner. If the publication is published by a nonprofit organization, give its name and address.)

Full Name	Complete Mailing Address
WHOLLY OWNED SUBSIDIARY OF REED/ELSEVIER, US HOLDINGS	1600 JOHN F KENNEDY BLVD. SUITE 1600 PHILADELPHIA, PA 19103-2899

11. Known Bondholders, Mortgagees, and Other Security Holders Owning or Holding 1 Percent or More of Total Amount of Bonds, Mortgages, or Other Securities. If none, check box. ▶ ☐ None

Full Name	Complete Mailing Address
N/A	

12. Tax Status (For completion by nonprofit organizations authorized to mail at nonprofit rates) (Check one)
The purpose, function, and nonprofit status of this organization and the exempt status for federal income tax purposes:
☒ Has Not Changed During Preceding 12 Months
☐ Has Changed During Preceding 12 Months (Publisher must submit explanation of change with this statement)

PS Form 3526, July 2014 (Page 1 of 4 (see instructions page 4)) PSN: 7530-01-000-9931   PRIVACY NOTICE: See our privacy policy on www.usps.com.

---

13. Publication Title	14. Issue Date for Circulation Data Below
FOOT AND ANKLE CLINICS OF NORTH AMERICA	MAY 2023

15. Extent and Nature of Circulation			Average No. Copies Each Issue During Preceding 12 Months	No. Copies of Single Issue Published Nearest to Filing Date
a. Total Number of Copies (Net press run)			202	201
b. Paid Circulation (By Mail and Outside the Mail)	(1)	Mailed Outside-County Paid Subscriptions Stated on PS Form 3541 (Include paid distribution above nominal rate, advertiser's proof copies, and exchange copies)	125	112
	(2)	Mailed In-County Paid Subscriptions Stated on PS Form 3541 (Include paid distribution above nominal rate, advertiser's proof copies, and exchange copies)	0	0
	(3)	Paid Distribution Outside the Mails Including Sales Through Dealers and Carriers, Street Vendors, Counter Sales, and Other Paid Distribution Outside USPS®	75	86
	(4)	Paid Distribution by Other Classes of Mail Through the USPS (e.g. First-Class Mail®)	1	2
c. Total Paid Distribution (Sum of 15b (1), (2), (3), and (4))		▶	201	200
d. Free or Nominal Rate Distribution (By Mail and Outside the Mail)	(1)	Free or Nominal Rate Outside-County Copies included on PS Form 3541	0	0
	(2)	Free or Nominal Rate In-County Copies Included on PS Form 3541	0	0
	(3)	Free or Nominal Rate Copies Mailed at Other Classes Through the USPS (e.g. First-Class Mail)	0	0
	(4)	Free or Nominal Rate Distribution Outside the Mail (Carriers or other means)	1	1
e. Total Free or Nominal Rate Distribution (Sum of 15d (1), (2), (3) and (4))		▶	1	1
f. Total Distribution (Sum of 15c and 15e)		▶	202	201
g. Copies not Distributed (See Instructions to Publishers #4 (page #3))		▶	0	0
h. Total (Sum of 15f and g)		▶	202	201
i. Percent Paid (15c divided by 15f times 100)			99.5%	99.5%

* If you are claiming electronic copies, go to line 16 on page 3. If you are not claiming electronic copies, skip to line 17 on page 3.

16. Electronic Copy Circulation		Average No. Copies Each Issue During Preceding 12 Months	No. Copies of Single Issue Published Nearest to Filing Date
a. Paid Electronic Copies	▶		
b. Total Paid Print Copies (Line 15c) + Paid Electronic Copies (Line 16a)	▶		
c. Total Print Distribution (Line 15f) + Paid Electronic Copies (Line 16a)	▶		
d. Percent Paid (Both Print & Electronic Copies) (16b divided by 16c × 100)	▶		

☒ I certify that 50% of all my distributed copies (electronic and print) are paid above a nominal price.

17. Publication of Statement of Ownership

☒ If the publication is a general publication, publication of this statement is required. Will be printed in the DECEMBER 2023 issue of this publication.   ☐ Publication not required.

18. Signature and Title of Editor, Publisher, Business Manager, or Owner

Malathi Samayan - Distribution Controller

Malathi Samayan   Date 9/18/2023

I certify that all information furnished on this form is true and complete. I understand that anyone who furnishes false or misleading information on this form or who omits material or information requested on the form may be subject to criminal sanctions (including fines and imprisonment) and/or civil sanctions (including civil penalties).

PS Form 3526, July 2014 (Page 2 of 4)   PRIVACY NOTICE: See our privacy policy on www.usps.com.

Moving?

Make sure your subscription moves with you!

To notify us of your new address, find your **Clinics Account Number** (located on your mailing label above your name), and contact customer service at:

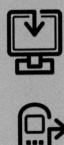

Email: journalscustomerservice-usa@elsevier.com

800-654-2452 (subscribers in the U.S. & Canada)
314-447-8871 (subscribers outside of the U.S. & Canada)

Fax number: 314-447-8029

Elsevier Health Sciences Division
Subscription Customer Service
3251 Riverport Lane
Maryland Heights, MO 63043

*To ensure uninterrupted delivery of your subscription, please notify us at least 4 weeks in advance of move.